I0489435

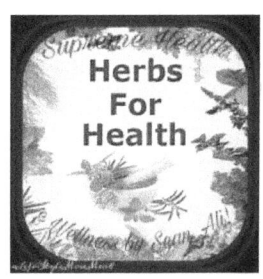

Herbs
For
Health

Understanding &
Creating Herbal
Healing!

Teas, Decoctions, Infusions & Tinctures!

Scientific Staff:	Kareem Tyree	Gabriella Monique
	Khalil Malik	

Supreme Health & Wellness by Sean Ali!

Achieving and Maintaining Supreme Health by increasing the level of Knowledge and Science of Life!

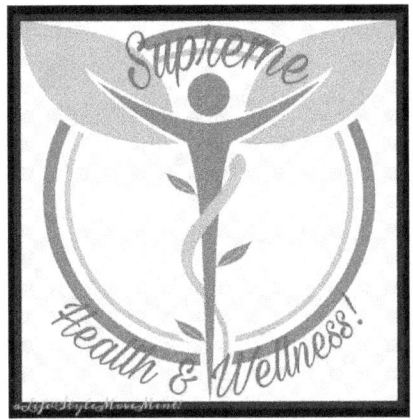

Dedicated to my Awesome FAMILY!

Table of Contents

****

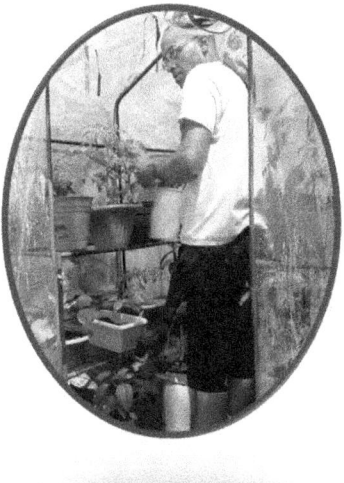

Introduction

❋❋❋❋❋

Peace and Blessings of Health!

This handbook represents Volume 2 of my Science Of Healing Series......as well as my Humble endeavor of collecting the best scientific research on naturally occurring Life & Healing Herbal Elements so that we can regain our Natural ability to Heal OurSelves!

In this Volume, the focus is on creating Teas, Decoctions and Tinctures, as well as the best research and recommendations on Dosages. This Handbook is designed to function as a handy pocket travel edition of Healing so that you can always have a quick reference available.

I must start with a note that we must understand that the ONLY reasons we get 'sick' or suffer from a 'dis-ease' is because of our mis-use or lack of performance of 1 of our 3 Life Functions - Respiration, Hydration and Energy Intake/Eating. There are certain dis-eases or conditions that can only occur through direct abuse of one of the above Life Functions and it is at this point or condition that we need Earth-based Solutions.

We come from the Earth and ALL our Solutions come from the Earth.......All we have to do is simply turn back to Mother Earth and extract what we Need!!!

It must also be understood that unless the behavior that lead to the dis-ease or condition – NOTHING will truly Help because the CAUSE will continue to produce the EFFECT!!!!

Many Dis-eases, conditions present with the same few underlying symptoms, with PAIN being the main identifying factor. Most Herbal Elements and/or Remedies were used to treat the Pain and discomfort to allow the Body to have the Energy and Focus to Heal.

With this being said, there are no Miracle Herbal Elements or Remedies that can instantly or 'magically' Heal instantly. Unfortunately, Life or the Healing process doesn't function like that. Almost every dis-ease or condition takes time to develop and the Healing process takes time as well.

This is why Herbal Elements were mainly used to Relieve pain, discomfort and Energy imbalances that were preventing the Body from creating the environment of Healing within itself.

We Come From The Earth …..And ALL Our Solutions Come From The Earth!

There are several symptoms and dis-eases that can be prevented, controlled or solved with Herbal Elements that are Naturally occurring and abundant on the Earth. In fact, many of these Herbal Life Elements we walk past everyday. Several we disregard or try to eradicate because they have been classified as 'weeds', not knowing that we are disregarding or trying to eliminate a Valuable Herbal Life Element.

In a time of Emergency this small Handbook could very well be the catalyst for Your Own personal Well-being and Survival.

For those of us that prefer to use our own God-Given intelligence and Abilities to turn back to the Earth and extract what we need, may this small Handbook be a Guide and/or Reference so that you can discover these Wonderful Naturally occurring Herbal Life Elements that may be right outside your door.

We Come From The Earth And ALL Our Solutions Come From the Earth........All We Have To DO Is Simply Turn Back To The Earth And Exract What We NEED!!!!

Achieving and Maintaining Supreme Health and Fitness by increasing the level of Knowledge and Science of LIFE!

PEACE!

Sean Ali

Supreme Health & Fitness

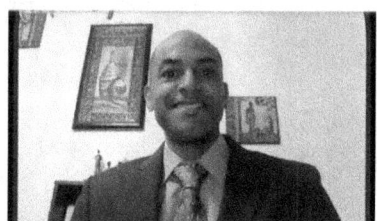

Create Your Healthy LifeStyle Now!

Wellness Programs for Your Abundant Life!
Open today until 10:00 PM

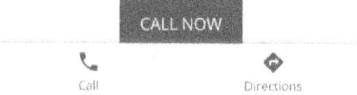

One

History of Herbal Healing

******

Herbal Elements are simply the Plant-life of the Earth, the same Earth that we come from and must turn to for all our Solutions. These Plants have been used by humans for food, medicine, clothing, and tools, as well as in religious rites every since we have populated our planet.

There are Catalogues of Herbal remedies in pharmacopoeias that date back 5000 years.

No continent, island, climate, or geography that is home to human culture lacks a formal tradition of incorporating local flora into daily and ceremonial life that was used as a means of enhancing health and well-being.

Unfortunately, only recently have many Western health care providers recognized the number of remedies that had their origin in Herbal medicine, with little still willing to accept or utilize these Ancient, successful Herbal remedies.

Fortunately, these Herbal remedies and products have gained increasing popularity in the last decade. When inquired, approximately ¼ of adults reported using an Herbal remedy to treat a medical illness within the past year.

The most common Herbal elements that were used included Ginkgo, Echinacea, Garlic, St. John's wort, Soy, Kava and Saw Palmetto. The global market for Herbal products exceeds over $60 billion annually.

In some instances the Native/Indigenous people also adopted "big medicine" from European "**physick**" and some early surgical practices as well, from the early Spanish conquistador Cabeza de Vaca, (1530), which eventually led to them taking the French word for physician *(médecin)* and incorporating it into their own languages to express something previously unknown.

Europeans were in turn impressed by Native American resort to the healing power of nature and to spiritual healing. Nature in the New World provided a bounty of new medicinal plants and foods (whereas in Europe there had been only 16 cultivars—before chocolate, corn, squash, tomatoes, peppers, potatoes, and other foods of the Americas).

In the English colonies beginning at Jamestown, (1607) Herbal Elements, such as *sassafras*, were readily adopted. In Pennsylvania, William Penn, (1680) himself became well acquainted with native herbal elements and other healing-spiritual practices such as the sweat lodge of the Delaware Natives.

Many of the earliest books to come out of the English colonies were natural histories, serving as "*herbals*," which documented the occurrence of medicinal plants found throughout various parts of the colonies. These regions are very bio-diverse with many plant species that have awesome healing and medicinal properties.

Physicians were rare on the expanding frontier, which prevented "regular medicine" (such as bleeding by lancet, leeches, and cupping; and blistering, puking, and purging—of which Francis Bacon had said, "The remedy is worse than the disease") from taking root and replacing the effective natural and home remedies already in-place.

The American "self-help" book first took hold on the frontier with the publication in 1734 of *Every Man His Own Doctor, Or, The Poor Planter's Physician* by John Tennent of rural Spotsylvania County, Virginia, describing many Native/Indigenous herbal remedies.

*The potent American **ginseng** of Appalachia quickly became an international commodity with exportation to China.* Frontiersman Daniel Boone for a time earned a living as a "**sanger**," which is the gathering of herbal elements in the wild.

In 1774, the leading American physician during this time, Benjamin Rush, published a treatise on the importance of Native American remedies. Amazingly for that era only one man died on the expedition, which lends proof that Nature was/is a healthier place than Civilization.

The "***west cure, rest cure, and nature cures***" became the recommended means of recuperating from the harsh illnesses of 19th century European civilization.

By the middle of the 19th century, the natural remedies of frontier medicine represented a well-established and widely available form of health care in America. During the Civil War, after the Union naval blockade of the South began working in 1862, the Confederacy found it difficult to obtain ***manufactured medicines*** and turned to ***natural remedies***, even publishing a pamphlet listing the native herbal elements that could be used for treatment. Some of these herbal elements included: ***snakeroot, sassafras, partridgeberry, lavender, dogwood, tulip tree, red*** and ***white oak***. Even the Confederate Medical Corps kits contained many of these remedies toward the end of the war.

After the Civil War introduced the beginning of patent (herbal) remedies, including Dr. Pepper, Dr. John Pemberton's Coca-Cola, and Dr. Hire's Root Beer, still enormously popular today as "soda," "pop," "tonic," and "root beer."

Also the derogatory term ***quacks*** (from the German word ***quacksalver*** "**quicksilver**" or "**mercury**," which was actually a toxic regular medical treatment of the time) began to be applied to the **practitioners** of natural remedies (who were coincidentally considered useful on the American frontier from the 1500s to the 1850s).

This demeaning term became in use suddenly at about the SAME time that the **American Medical Association** was organized in 1847 in reaction to and in opposition to the formation of the **American Homeopathic Association** in 1842.

Physicians and scientists who made real health advances with the use of natural healing in the mid- to late 19th century (Thomson; Vincent Priessnitz [the *water* cure]; Russell Trall [the *nature* cure]; Nikola Tesla, pioneer of *electromagnetism*) were rounded up in the judgment of 20th century history together with **true** quacks/charlatans like Thomas Alva Edison, Jr. (son of the inventor, who did his best to put the true genius of electricity and bio-energy - Tesla, out of business), John Romulus Brinkley, Dr. C. Everett Field, and Norman Baker.

This label of 'quack' also came to be applied to hypnotists and "magnetic" healers (e.g., Franz Anton Mesmer) and the emerging manual therapists (e.g., Andrew Taylor Still, Daniel David Palmer) of the 19th century who originated in and were also initially a phenomenon of the rural frontier.

For several decades many have awaited the next "miracle" drug, biotech breakthrough, and, now, medical information technology for solutions to our health care crisis.

This book illustrates that often it is ancient knowledge and wisdom about healing that, when adapted to new circumstances, provide truly innovative approaches to health problems.

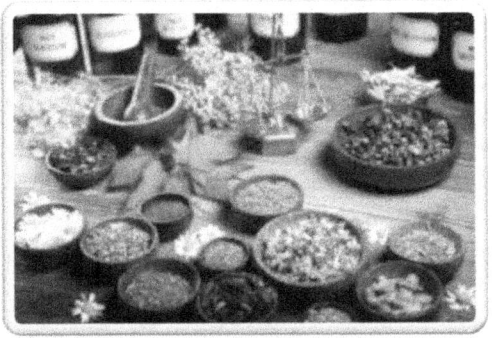

Two

Understanding the Herbal Elements

*****

The word *Herb* as a word has an ancient pedigree that originates with the Latin word *Herba*, which refers to *green crops* and *grasses* and could also mean the same as we mean by *Herb* today (Oxford English Dictionary, or OED). The word entered English through Old French, with the English use of "*herb*" in the sense of a plant whose stem *does not* become woody and persistent but remains more-or-less *soft* and *succulent*, while dying down to the ground (or entirely) after flowering, can be traced to the thirteenth century. In the 13th century it was also understood that an "*Herb*" (with variant spellings, e.g., "*erbe*") is a plant whose leaves and stems (and sometimes roots) could be used as *food* or *medicine* or for *scent* or *flavor.*

Herbarium, is defined in the sense of a collection of dried plants and has its origins in the 18th century. A source for the definition of "*herbarium*" dealing with the medicinal properties of plants is developed on the claim that the science of drying plants for study originated with a professor in Italy in the 16th century who also held a chair in "simples," in which he studied medicinal and other plants.

The term *Herbalist* has shifted meaning. Originally beginning in the 16th century, an "*herbalist*" was one knowledgeable in the us *herbs* and *plants*—a collector of and writer about plants, which would describe what we mean by "*botanist*" today.

Usually a "*herbalist*" is now used to refer to early writers about plants, as well as persons who use alternative medical therapy, although the OED does not mention this.

The term *Herbal* is defined as a book containing names and descriptions of herbs (or other plants in general) that provides properties and virtues came into use in the early sixteenth century. "*Herbal*" meaning belonging to, consisting of, or made from *herbs* and has its origins in the early 17th century.

The term *Medical Botany* is the study of the medicinal properties of plants, an example is a chemical analysis to find new medically important compounds. A medical botanical garden would be the source of plants for studying their medical properties.

A *Medicinal Herb Garden* is technically a place that has examples of plants, from which samples could be taken to make medicinal preparations. Also, the garden would contain only herbaceous plants, not plants with woody stems and branches

Herbalism is the *study* and *practice* of using plant material for food, medicine, and health promotion. This science includes not only *treatment* of disease but also *enhancement* of quality of life, both physically and spiritually. A fundamental principle of herbalism is to promote preventive care and guided, simple treatment for the general population. An *Herbalist*, or *Herbal Practitioner*, is someone who has undertaken specific study and supervised practical training to achieve competence in treating patients. *Herbal Medicines* are recommended by physicians in the practice of integrative medicine and by other practitioners within the pharmacopeia of their tradition.

Herbal & Medicinal Elements

*****

Physicians in the United States studied and relied on plant drugs as primary medicines through the 1930s until World War II. Until then, medical schools taught basic plant taxonomy and **pharmacognosy** and medicinal plant therapeutics.

The term *drug* derives from an ancient word for *root*, and the roots and rhizomes of many medicinal plants continue to provide alkaloids, steroidal saponins, and many active constituents that are clinically useful today.

The *United States Pharmacopeia* listed 636 herbal entries in 1870; only 58 were listed in the 1990 edition (Boyle, 1991). Although some plants were dropped because they were found to be weak or unsafe, the majority of clinically useful plants were replaced with pharmaceuticals, which generated profits from patented drugs and contributed to the standardization and industrialization of medicine.

Food, medicinal, and healing plants may contain *digestible fiber* (carbohydrates and hemicellulose) and *indigestible fiber* (cellulose and lignin's), *nutritive* (calories, vitamins, minerals, trace elements, amino acids, essential fatty acids, and water), and *inert* and *active* constituents.

Herbal Practices:

*****

Herbal Practitioners normally rely on one of the following, or a combination:

1.   *The plant's pharmacological actions:* in some cases enhanced by specific processing and extractive solvents and techniques or formulation of plant medicines into standardized extract products to concentrate and guarantee unit doses of active constituents

2.   *Individual plant pharmacokinetics:* best preserved by using single, whole plants or their extracts

3.   *Synergistic formulating:* is the blending of a number of medicinal plants together to achieve specific therapeutic effects unachievable by using a single herb alone

4.   *Nutritional value:* as when *Urtica repens,* or nettles, is recommended as a tea rich in absorbable iron

5.   *Energetics:* Vibrational energy, as for example with Bach Flower remedies, and various flower essences.

Herbal Therapeutics:

*****

Herbal medicines can be delivered in many forms. Some plants are best when used fresh but are seldom marketed fresh because they are highly perishable, and improper storage will affect quality. Dried, whole, or chopped herbal elements can be prepared either as *infusions* (steeped as tea) or *decoctions* (simmered over low heat).

Typically, flowers, leaves, and powdered herbs are **infused** (e.g., chamomile or peppermint), whereas fruits, seeds, barks, and roots require **decocting** (e.g., rose hips, cinnamon bark, licorice root).

Many *fresh* and *dried herbs* can be **tinctured** as medicines preserved in alcohol. Some plants are suited to **acetracts** (vinegar extracts), whereas others are active and well preserved as **syrups**, **glycerides** (in vegetable glycerine), or **miels** (in honey).

Powered or *freeze-dried* herbal elements are available in bulk and as tablets, troches, pastes, and capsules.

Fluid and *solid extracts*—strong concentrates (four to six times the crude herb strength)—and fresh plant juices preserved in approximately 25% alcohol (as with the fresh plant *Echinacea succus*) are other forms.

Non-oral delivery forms include *herbal pessaries, suppositories, creams, ointments, gels, liniments, oils, distilled waters, washes, enemas, baths, poultices, compresses, moxa, snuffs, steams*, and *inhaled smokes* and *aromatics* (volatile oils).

Capsules and *tablets* are the most common delivery system. Gelatin or vegetable-based **capsules** are filled with powdered dried herbs. Tablets are powdered herbal elements compressed into a solid pill, often with a variety of inert ingredients as fillers.

Herbal Elements are supplied in a variety of sizes and strengths, so it is important to read the label *carefully*. The label also usually gives an average suggested dose as a guideline, based on research and clinical use. It is also recommended to start at the *low end*; watch for a response, including unwanted effects; and adjust the dose accordingly.

General Guidelines for Use of Herbal Medicines:

*****

1.   The clinician should take a careful history of the patient's use of herbal elements and other supplements.

2.   An accurate medical diagnosis must be made before herbal elements are used for symptomatic treatment.

3.   *Natural* is not necessarily *safe;* attention should be paid to quality of product, dosage, and potential adverse effects, including interactions.

4.   Herbal treatments should, for the most part, be avoided in pregnancy (and contemplated pregnancy) and lactation.

5.   Herbal use by children should be done with care, using the appropriate dosage based on weight.

6.   Adverse effects should be recorded, and the dosage reduced or the product discontinued. It can be carefully restarted to ascertain whether or not it is the source of the problem.

Herbal Life Elements Classifications

*****

The Science of how Herbal Elements are classified is just as vital and should be a main focus and taught simultaneously with Knowing the type and name of the Herb.

Knowing the Class of a particular Herbal Element allows for proper use as well as avoiding any potential life/health threatening issues. This is especially important since 90% of all pharmaceuticals are Herbal Elements based.

The *American Herbal Products Association* (AHPA) created a rating system that classifies Herbal Element products according to their relative safety and potential toxicity based on the following four categories:

<u>Class 1</u> : Herbal elements that can be consumed safely when used appropriately.

<u>Class 2</u> : Herbal elements for which the following use restrictions apply, unless otherwise directed by an expert qualified in the use of the described substance:

2a - For external use only.

2b - Not to be used during pregnancy.

2c - Not to be used while nursing.

2d - Other specific use restrictions as noted.

Class 3 : Herbs for which sufficient research exists to recommend the Herbal Element to be addressed with the following labeling: "<u>**To be used only under the supervision of an expert qualified in the appropriate use of this substance**</u>."

Labeling must include proper use information as follows: dosage, contraindications, potential adverse effects and drug interactions, and any other relevant information related to the safe use of the substance.

Class 4 : Herbal elements for which insufficient data are available for classification.

Active Chemical Constituents in Plants

*****

1. *Carbohydrates*: sugars, starches, aldehydes, gums, and pectin's

2. *Glycosides*: cardiac glycosides in *Digitalis purpureal* leaf, anthraquinone glycosides in *Aloe* species latex and rhubarb *(Rheum officinale)* root and rhizome, flavanol glycosides (rutin and hesperidin, used to reduce capillary bleeding), and other glycoside types

3. *Tannins*: present in coffee and tea

4. *Lipids*: fixed oils and waxes

5. *Volatile oils*: essential oils such as peppermint and eucalyptus

6. *Resins*

7. *Steroids*: including the steroidal saponins from Mexican yam *(Diocorea* species), the original source of early oral contraceptives

8. *Alkaloids*: atropine from *Atropa belladonna*, quinine from cinchona, morphine from *Papaver somniferum*

9. *Peptide hormones*

10. *Enzymes*: bromelain from pineapple.

Safety & Precautions

*****

Side effects of drugs can be serious or fatal; the worst is death by overdose. According to one report, overdoses are associated with an annual rate of 30.1 deaths per 1 million prescriptions of antidepressants. On the other hand, to quote Norman Farnsworth, PhD, professor of pharmacognosy at the University of Illinois, Chicago, "Based on published reports, side effects or toxic reactions associated with herbal medicines in any form are rare.... In fact, of all classes of substances ... to cause toxicities of sufficient magnitude to be reported in the United States, plants are the least problematic."

Herbal products are often **considered safe** because they are "**natural**" products (Kuruvilla, 2002). Nonetheless, the quality of products may be affected by species differences, seasonal variations, environmental factors, collection methods, transport and storage, manufacturing practices, or contamination with foreign plant material, toxins, heavy metals, or environmental pollutants.

One must also remember that any substance that has biological activity has the potential to cause adverse effects. Dangerous and lethal side effects related to direct toxic effects, allergic reactions, effects from contaminants, and interaction with drugs or other **herbs** have been reported, (Chan, 2003; Dobos et al, 2005; Hu et al, 2005; Izzo et al, 2001).

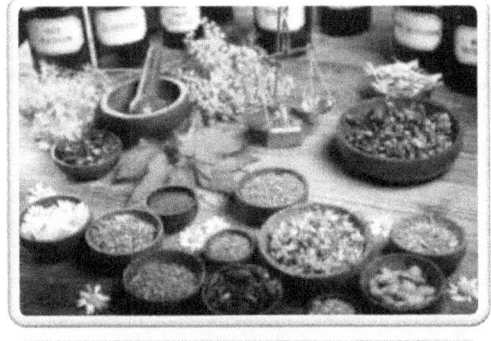

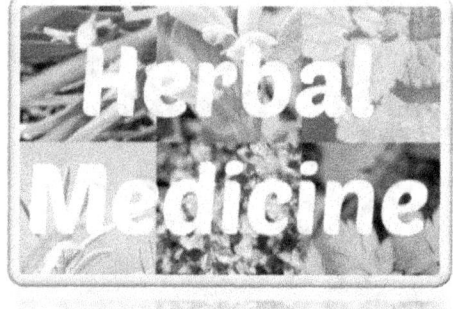

Three

Dosages, Teas, Infusions, Decoctions & Tinctures!

*****

Dos·age
['dōsij]

Noun:

Dosages (plural noun)

1. the size or frequency of a **dose** of a medicine or drug:

- a level of exposure to or absorption of ionizing radiation.

Dosage Guidelines:

These Herbal Life Elements are considered **medicinal** and as with any Medicine, proper handling must be ensured. Always Start with the *lowest dose* in the range and work up.

Frequency and Consistency: 1 large dose per day is not as effective as **3-4** **small doses.**

Tea

[tē]

*****

Origin:

Mid 17th cent.: probably via Malay from Chinese (Min dialect) te; related to Mandarin chá.

Noun:

1. a hot drink made by infusing the dried, crushed leaves of the tea plant in boiling water.

- the dried leaves used to make tea.

- a hot drink made from the infused leaves, fruits, or flowers of other plants.

2. the Evergreen shrub or small tree that produces tea leaves, native to South and eastern Asia and grown as a major cash crop.

*****

How to Make Herbal Teas:

- **1 cup** boiling water

- **1 tsp** *dried* or **2-3 tsp** *fresh* leaves, stems, or flowers

Steep together **3-5 min** in a covered pot; strain; serve the liquid Tea when temperature is appropriate.

*****

Tea Dosage Guidelines:

Age of Child	Dosage
<1 yrs	1 tsp daily, working up to 1 tsp tid
1-2 yrs	1 oz-¼ cup daily, working up to ¼ cup tid
3-6 yrs	¼-½ cup daily, working up to tid
7-11 yrs	Up to 6 oz daily, working up to tid-qid
12 yrs-adult	1 cup daily, working up to tid-qid

De·coc·tion

[dəˈkäkSH(ə)n]

*****

Origin:

Late Middle English: from late Latin decoctio(n-), from **decoquere** 'boil down'

Noun:

Decoctions (plural noun)

1. the liquor resulting from concentrating the essence of a substance by heating or boiling, especially a medicinal preparation made from a plant.

2. the action or process of extracting the essence of something.

Herbal **Teas** and **Decoctions** are very similar in preparations and both can be very pleasurable to drink, but can also, with regular use, **tone**, **soothe**, and **balance** the body.

We use the **Decoction** method of brewing **tea** when working with the **hard**, **woody** substances (such as roots, bark, and stems) that have constituents that are water-soluble and non-volatile.

A versatile form, a decoction can be drunk on their own, made into syrups, honeys, gargles, compresses, and douches or added to baths.

It can also be incorporated into oils and creams.

<u>Understanding the Decoction method:</u>

In addition to the traditional recipe for brewing **tea** (**1-cup boiling water** poured over **1-t dried herbal element** or **2-t fresh herb**), you may also choose to make an **infusion** (which is stronger than a tea) or a **decoction**.

- The **decoction** method is used for **hard, woody** substances (such as roots, bark, and stems) that have constituents that are water-soluble and non-volatile. (Red clover is an exception, because red clover flower **decoction** will extract more minerals that the infusion.)

- **Decoctions** extract mainly **mineral salts** and **bitter principles**. **Decoctions** are intended for **immediate use**.

- Store for a maximum of **72 hours** in the refrigerator.

******

<u>Light Decoction</u>

- This method is used for such lighter barks as willow or cinnamon and some hard leaves like horsetail or horehound.
- Make a decoction by simmering the herbs, covered, on the lowest heat possible for ten to fifteen minutes.
- Leaving the lid on the pot prevents the escape of volatile constituents like essential oils.
- Let the mixture steep for another ten or fifteen minutes, then strain and use or refrigerate

Reduced Decoction

- This method is used for expensive herbs.
- After the first simmering, strain the herbs and set the strained liquid aside.
- Add more fresh water to the herbs, but only about one-quarter the amount used in the first simmering.
- Simmer for thirty minutes.
- Let cool for fifteen minutes and strain, squeezing out as much liquid as possible from the herbs.
- Blend the two liquid extractions together. A third simmering is not productive as the first two are able to obtain more than 90% of the medicinal constituents from the herb.

*****

Maceration

- 25 g herb
- 500 ml cold, filtered water
- Pour the water over the herb and let stand overnight.
- Strain and use like a decoction.
- Since heat destroys the active components of some herbs, a cold maceration is more appropriate than a decoction.

How to Make Herbal Decoctions:

- 2 tsp *dried* herb **or** up to 6 tsp *fresh* herb
- 2 cups water

1. Combine and simmer gently 5-15 min; strain; cool before serving the liquid.

2. Place the water into a pot made from **non-reactive metal** (such as **stainless** or **enamel**; <u>do not use aluminum</u>).

3. Cut or crush the herbal element or root and add it to the water in the pot. (<u>**Do not cut or crush the herbal element or root in advance, as vital constituents can be lost**</u>.)

4. Turn the heat to medium. Simmer your **decoction** with the lid off until the **volume** of water is reduced by **one-quarter** (so, three-quarters of a pint remains).

5. Cool and strain. Store in the fridge for no more than 72 hours.

Use a **decoction** when an herbal element is better simmered than steeped to extract their specific Life Energy/Nutrients. For an example, oat-straw contains silica, which requires simmering to be released into the water.

In·fu·sion

{in'fyo͞oZHən}

*****

Origin:

From Latin **infusio**(n-), from the verb **infundere**. Late Middle English (denoting the pouring in of a liquid):

Noun

noun: **infusion**; plural noun: **infusions**

1. a drink, remedy, or extract prepared by soaking the leaves of a plant or herb in liquid.
   a. the process of preparing an extract by soaking the leaves of a plant in liquid.
2. the introduction of a new element or quality into something.
3. Medicine .... the slow injection of a substance into a vein or tissue.

Herbal infusions have been used for thousands of years. Many of us create them regularly when we **brew tea** (which is simply an infusion of tea leaves).

When deciding whether to prepare an herbal infusion or a **decoction**, consider what nutritional goals you hope to achieve.

Are you looking to **support a healthy body and mind**? Or maybe you just want a deliciously nourishing beverage that is different from your everyday drink!

The answer will determine not just what herbs you use, but also the method you use to make the most of them.

Hot Herbal Infusions

Hot infusions draw out vitamins, enzymes, and aromatic volatile oils. **Flowers, leaves, and aromatic roots** are all ideal ingredients for hot infusions. Some examples include **ginger root**, **nettle leaf**, **holy basil**, **red clover**, **horsetail**, and **raspberry leaf**, just to list a few!

Nutrient-rich herbs add an extra dimension to your daily regimen and work synergistically to support overall health. There is an abundance of options when creating combinations for hot infusions, offering an excellent opportunity to tap into your creative side.

Steep time will depend on your personal flavor preferences and the specific herbs used.

The longer certain herbs are steeped, the stronger their flavors.

Different nutritional benefits are also gained from different steep times for specific herbs, as longer steeping times tend to draw out more minerals.

Generally, you'll want to steep herbs for longer than you would black, green, or white **tea leaves**.

How to make a Hot Infusion

Directions

1. Scoop 1 to 3 tablespoons of **dried herbs** into a **tea strainer** placed in your **teapot** or **mug**.
2. Heat water until it just comes to a boil.
3. Pour hot water over herbs to submerge them and cover to help hold in any volatile oils.
4. Steep for 15 minutes to 1 hour and strain.

*****

Cold Herbal Infusions

Cold infusions are ideal for enjoying the benefits of **mucilaginous herbs** and herbs with delicate essential oils.

A few good herbs for cold infusions include **marshmallow root, peppermint leaf, rose buds**, or freshly harvested herbs such as lemon balm or St. John's Wort.

Since there is no boiling involved in this preparation, bacteria growth can happen more quickly than with hot infusions.

Be sure to use clean tools, refrigerate your infusion if you're not going to drink it right away, and consume or dispose of it within a week (or sooner if you notice an off taste, smell, or change in appearance).

*****

How To Make a Cold Infusion

Directions

1. Fill a quart jar with cold water.
2. Bundle 1 ounce of herb in **cheesecloth** or **muslin bag**.
3. Slightly moisten the herb inside the bundle (for easier submersion.)
4. Submerge the bundle just below the water in the jar.
5. Drape the tied end of the bundle over the lip of the jar.
6. Secure by loosely screwing on the cap.
7. Allow to infuse overnight.

Or

1. Place loose herbs in a quart jar, fill with cold water, and cap.
2. Allow to infuse overnight.
3. Strain herbs out with a **sprouting screen** and lid or **funnel with filter**.

Tinc·ture
[ˈtiNG(k)(t)SHər]
*****

Origin:

Late Middle English (denoting a dye or pigment): from Latin **tinctura** 'dyeing,' from **tingere** 'to dye or color.'

Noun:

Tinctures (plural noun)

      a. a medicine made by dissolving a drug in alcohol.

  2. **synonyms**: solution · suspension · infusion · elixir

      a. a slight trace of something.

      b. Heraldry;

  3. any of the conventional colors (including the metals and stains, and often the furs) used in coats of arms.

Verb:

Tinctured (past participle) · **tinctures** (third person present) · **tincturing** (present participle).

1. (be tinctured)

be tinged, flavored, or imbued with a slight amount of.

Tinctures are concentrated herbal extracts that are made using alcohol and chopped herbal elements.

The **tincture** is especially effective in drawing out the **essential compounds** of plants, especially those that are fibrous or woody, and from roots and resins.

Since this method ensures that the herbal elements and their Life Essence/Nutrients can be preserved for a long time, it is often mentioned in herbal books and remedies as a preferred way of using herbs.

In addition, many herbalists, including myself, love **tinctures** because they are easy to carry, they have a unique utility for long-term treatments, and their ability to be absorbed rapidly, as well as allowing for immediate dosage changes. It's easy to add juice to disguise the flavor as well should the **tincture** prove bitter.

Another benefit of **tinctures** is that they keep the Life Energy/Nutrients from the herbal elements in a stable, soluble form and they retain the volatile and semi-volatile ingredients that are otherwise lost in heat-treatment and processing of dry herbal extracts.

*****

What You Will Need:

- Mason jar(s) or other wide mouth jar with lid

- Unbleached muslin cloth

- Label / marker

- At least 80 proof vodka or other suitable alcohol

- Fresh or dried herb product, powdered or cut and sifted

How to Make an Herbal Tincture:

Prepare the tincture. It is best to prepare a **tincture** by measurement or by measured weight. Also, you should know whether you want to add fresh, powdered, or dried herbal elements to the **tincture**.

*****

Plant Material Proportions (Fresh vs. Dried)

Your first step is to fill your tincturing container with the correct amount of herbs. Proportions are important here: too little, and you'll end up with a weak tincture. Too much, and the amount of alcohol added won't be enough to pull out all the plant goodness from your herbs.

The **appropriate alcohol strength** and the relative amount of plant material to use will vary based on what you're tincturing.

*****

Here are some basic measurement guidelines:

Fresh Leaves and Flowers

- Finely chop or grind clean herb to release juice and expose surface area.
- Only fill jar 2/3 to 3/4 with herb.
- Pour alcohol to the very top of the jar. Cover plants completely!
- Jar should appear full of herb, but herb should move freely when shaken.

Dried Leaves and Flowers

- Use finely cut herbal material.
- Only fill jar 1/2 to 3/4 with herb.
- Pour alcohol to the very top of the jar. Cover plants completely!

*****

Fresh Roots, Barks & Berries

- Finely chop or grind clean plants to release juice and expose surface area.
- Only fill jar 1/3 to 1/2 with fresh roots, barks, or berries.
- Pour alcohol to the very top of the jar. Cover plants completely!
- Jar should appear full of herb, but herb should move freely when shaken.

*****

Dried Roots, Barks & Berries

- Use finely cut herbal material.
- Only fill jar 1/4 to 1/3 with dried roots, barks, or berries.
- Pour alcohol to the very top of the jar. Cover plants completely!
- Roots and berries will double in size when reconstituted!

Alcohol Type and Strength

Once you've filled your container with the correct amount of plant material, you'll need to fill the rest of the space with a high-proof alcohol. Most spirits will work, but many herbalists favor a high-quality, clear, and low-flavor liquor like vodka or grain alcohol.

Note that stronger alcohol types can be diluted with distilled water to reach a lower alcohol content by volume.

The appropriate alcohol strength for your tincture will depend upon the qualities of the plant material being used. Stronger is not always better!

Purchase quality alcohol. The preferred type of alcohol for producing a tincture is <u>vodka**</u> and the 'EverClear' brand is the best choice. This is owing to its being colorless, odorless, and almost flavorless. If you cannot obtain vodka, brandy, rum, or whiskey can be substituted.

Whatever alcohol is chosen, it must be **80 proof (40% alcohol)** to prevent mildewing of the plant material in the bottle.

- It is also possible to make a tincture from quality <u>apple cider vinegar</u> or quality vegetable glycerin.

- The alternatives may work better where the patient refuses alcohol.

Tips for matching Alcohol strength to Herbal Element:

40% to 50% alcohol by volume (80- to 90-proof vodka)

- "Standard" percentage range for tinctures.
- Good for most dried herbs and fresh herbs that are not super juicy.
- Good for extraction of water-soluble properties.

67.5% to 70% alcohol by volume (half 80-proof vodka and half 190-proof grain alcohol)

- Extracts the most volatile aromatic properties.
- For fresh, high-moisture herbs like lemon balm, berries, and aromatic roots.
- The higher alcohol percentage will draw out more of the plant juices.

85% to 95% alcohol by volume (190-proof grain alcohol)

- Good for dissolving gums and resins but not necessary for most plant material.
- Extracts the aromatics and essential oils bound in a plant that don't dissipate easily.
- This alcohol strength can produce a tincture that's not easy to take and will also dehydrate the herbs if used for botanicals beyond gums and resins.

** **Use a suitable container.** The container for the **tincture** should be glass or ceramic.

Avoid using metallic or plastic containers because these can react with the **tincture** or leach dangerous chemicals over time. Ensure that all containers are both washed clean and <u>sterilized</u> prior to use.

****

- *Add enough fresh chopped herbs to fill the glass container. Cover with alcohol.
- *Add 4 ounces (113g) of powdered herb with 1 pint (473ml) of alcohol (or vinegar/glycerin).
- *Add 7 ounces (198g) of dried herb material to 35 fluid ounces (1 liter) of alcohol (or vinegar/glycerin).

*****

Seal the container.

Place it into a cool, dark area; a cupboard shelf works best. The container should be stored there for 8 days to a month. It is common practice to let a **tincture** infuse for 6 weeks.

** Shake the container regularly. There is a difference on how often to shake the **tincture**. It is best practice to shake the bottle twice a week for the 1st two weeks. After that it can rest.

**Be sure to label the steeping tincture so that you know what it is and the date on which it was made. Keep it out of the reach of children and pets.

Strain the tincture.

Once the steeping time is finished (either the **tincture** instructions you're following will inform you of this or you'll know already from experience but if not, about two weeks is a good steeping time), strain the **tincture** as follows:

a. Place a muslin cloth across a sieve. Place a large bowl underneath to catch the strained liquid.

b. Gently pour the steeped liquid through the muslin-lined sieve. The muslin will capture the plant material and the liquid will pass through into the bowl underneath.

c. Press the herbal material with a wooden or bamboo spoon to squeeze out some more liquid, and lastly, twist the muslin to extract any leftover liquid from the herbal element.

Decant the liquid into a prepared tincture bottle.

Use a small funnel for this step if you don't have a steady hand. Tighten the lid and date and label the **tincture**.

If you're storing this for long-term without using until later, consider sealing the caps with wax.

Store and use.

A **tincture** can have a shelf life of up to 5 years owing to the fact that alcohol is a preservative.

Always know the properties of the particular herbal elements that you've used, and follow the guidance of the recipe from which you're making the **tincture** in terms of how long to keep the **tincture** for.

Follow the instructions relevant to your **tincture** for usage; consult a qualified, reputable herbalist or a health professional if you need more information and bear in mind that herbal treatments can be **dangerous** if you don't know the properties of the herbal element and its consequences.

*****

Tincture Dosage Guidelines:

Age of Child	Dosage
≤2 yrs	Not recommended for use
3-6 yrs	2-10 drops in ¼ cup water daily, working up to tid
7-11 yrs	10-20 drops in 6 oz water daily, working up to tid-qid
12 yrs-adult	20-50 drops up to tid-qid

*****

Warnings:

- High concentrations (about 40+%) are flammable so watch out if you are working near heat, or especially open flames.
- Keep out of the reach of children and pets.

- Some herbal remedies that are fine for the general population can be harmful for specific members of the population, such as infants, children, pregnant and breastfeeding women, and persons with lowered immune systems or allergies. Know the properties of the herbs and the possible complications of the patient!

- For dosing information - Again, if you don't know, consult your doctor or a qualified health professional before using.

- Always consult your doctor or a qualified health professional **before** using any herbal treatment. If you don't know what you're doing, then don't do it; get expert advice.

*****

Tips:

- It is cheaper to make your own tinctures than to buy them from a health store.

- A coffee filter can be used in place of the muslin cloth.

- Avoid using pots made of steel, iron, and any other metal. Some herbs react to them.

- Tinctures last longer than dried herbs, usually up to 2-5 years.

- You can "burn off" the alcohol by putting the dose into a cup of boiling water and drinking as a tea.

- You can make combinations of herbs if you have instructions to follow from a reputable source.

- You can control the quality of the herbal product in the tincture by making adjustments; follow the tincture instructions.

*****

A to Z ~ Herbal Elements

*****

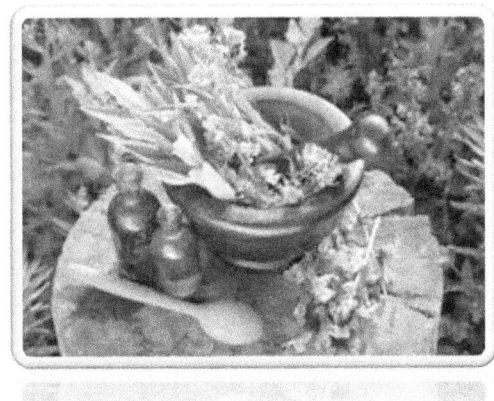

Glossary of Herbs
by Plant Parts

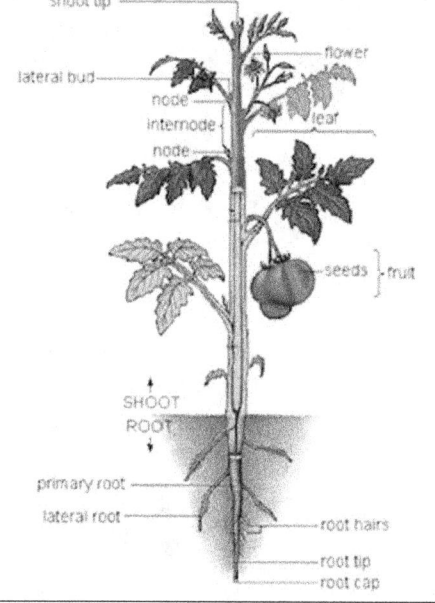

Aloe:

Uses: Topical treatment of minor burns, sunburn, cuts, abrasions, insect bites, acne, poison ivy, frostbite, itching of chicken pox.

***Not recommended for internal use in children. Decreased bowel transit time reduces absorption of other medications.

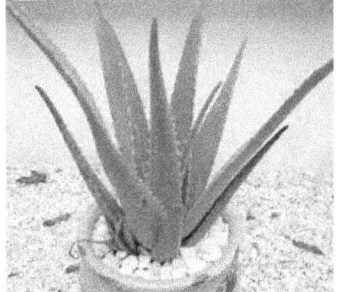

Research/Future Possibilities: Changes in chemical composition of urine after Aloe gel consumption show potential for preventing kidney-stone formation among children.

Precautions: For **external** use only in children <12 yrs

Dosage/Administration:

◊ **Topical**: break off leaf, split lengthwise, apply gel to affected skin.

*****

Angelica Archangelica:

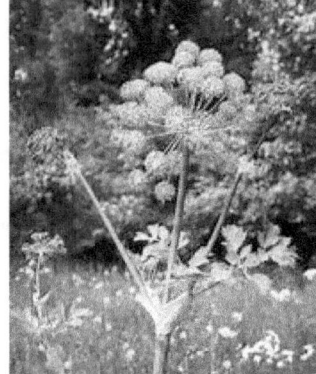

Uses: Relaxing expectorant, diaphoretic, carminative, diuretic

Precautions: Avoid during pregnancy.

Dosage/Administration:

◇ **Tea**: Simmer **1 tablespoon** of root pieces in 2 cups of boiling water for 15 minutes. Cover while simmering. Take 1 tablespoon to ½ cup up to every 4 hours.

◇ **Tincture**: **10-40 drops** up to every 4 hours.

Anise:

Uses: Cough, expectorant, colic

Research: Anise oil exhibited a high level of antiviral activity against acyclovir-sensitive herpes simplex type 1

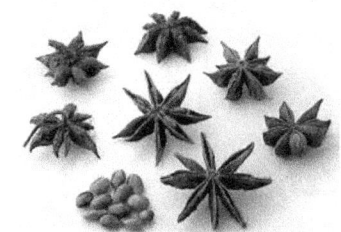

Precautions: Do not give the essential oil to children.

Dosage/Administration

⋄   **Decoct 1 tsp** seed in 1 cup water; strain and serve several times/day,

⋄   **Tea**: PO: ½-3 cups daily

⋄   **Tincture**: **5 drops** up to 4 times in 1 hour for colic; ¼-½ tsp up to every 4 hours

*****

Astragalus

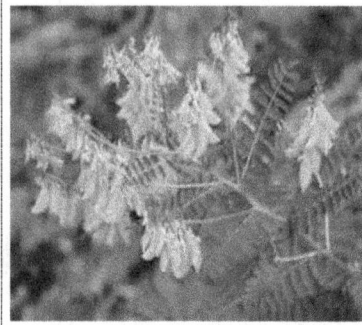

Uses: Immune system support

Precautions: Do not use during fevers; use only *Astragalus membranaceus* sp.; do not use wild species of American astragalus.

Dosage/Administration:

◇   **Capsules/extract**: follow package directions

◇   **Cooked**: drop **1 stick** of herbal element into cooking pot when making soup or cooked grains

◇   **Tea**: use **1 stick** of herb decocted in 1 cup water; see <u>tea dosage guidelines.</u>

◇   **Tincture**: ½–1 tsp 2–3 times/day.

Barberry:

Uses: Nausea, diarrhea, mucous conditions such as coughs

Precautions: At first, Barberry increases the amount of mucus being expelled, so start with small doses; do not take for more than 10 days at a time because extended consumption may decrease B-vitamin absorption and utilization; do not give barberry if the child has high blood pressure.

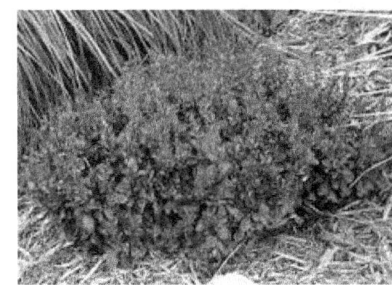

Dosage/Administration:

◊ **Extract** (strength of 1:1): use ⅛ **tsp** in 4 oz water, sipped slowly over an hour, (<u>Kemper, 1996</u>)

◊ **Tincture** (strength of 1:5): use **2-3 drops** in 4 oz water, sipped slowly over an hour, (<u>Kemper, 1996</u>).

*****

Benzoin

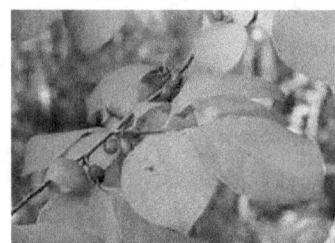

Uses: Topically as an antiseptic; as an inhalant and expectorant for bronchial disorders

Precautions: Allergy to benzoin can develop and cross-react with Mastisol; discontinue use if any hypersensitivity reactions occur, (James, 1984).

Dosage/Administration:

◊   **Inhalant**: 5 ml Benzoin gum/1 pt water; breathe vapors

◊   **Topical**: apply to affected area every 2-4 hrs; test a small area before applying to larger one.

Black Haw

Uses: Relieves muscle cramps or spasms, including irritable bladder muscles; menstrual pain

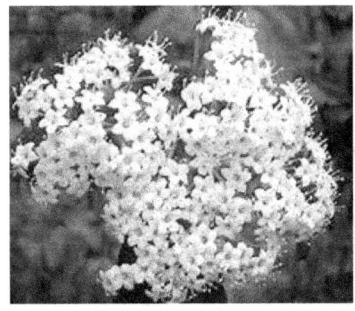

Precautions: Do not use if history of kidney stones or kidney disease

Dosage/Administration:

⋄   **Capsule/decoction**: for a 50-lb child (age approx 7 yrs) use ½ capsule or ½ cup decoction up to **qid**,

⋄   **Cream**: apply topically to relieve muscle cramps,

⋄   **Tea**: see tea dosage guidelines,

*****

Boneset

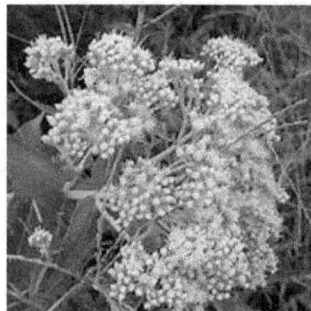

Uses: Colds and flu, to promote sweating, expectorant, antispasmodic

Precautions: High doses can cause vomiting; not for children <1 yr; do not administer for longer than 7 days; can cause contact dermatitis in those hypersensitive to Asteraceae,

Dosage/Administration:

➤ **Tea**: ¾ cup for 40-lb child, **tid** up to 3 days; adjust quantity by weight of child; better too little than too much,
➤ see tea dosage guidelines.

Burdock

Uses: Skin irritations, eczema, psoriasis

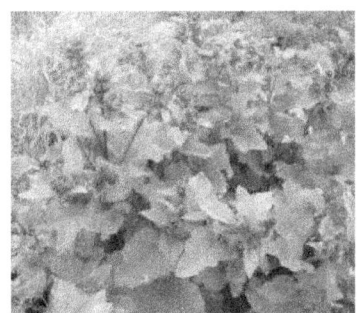

Precautions: Insulin dose may need to be adjusted because of hypoglycemic effect of Burdock, (Brinker, 1998); commercial sample may be adulterated with belladonna; do not give for longer than 2 wks; take a 1-wk break after a 2-wk regimen.

Dosage/Administration:

➤ **Capsule/tea**: **1 capsule**/day or 1 cup tea/day for a 50-lb child, (White, 1998);
➤ see tea dosage guidelines
➤ **Tincture**: ¼–½ tsp up to 4 times/day,

*****

Catnip

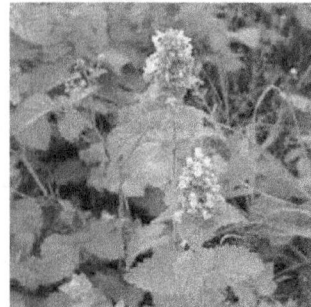

Uses: Colic, relaxes spasms and cramps, clears flatulence, sleeplessness, minor fevers

Precautions: None known when using a reasonable amount, (Vessey, 2001); there is a potential additive effect with drugs that sedate, such as anticonvulsants, antianxiety medications, and tricyclic antidepressants,

Dosage/Administration:

◇ **Tea** (internal): nursing mothers can take adult dose to ease baby's colic; a few oz daily for infants—can give in dropper alongside nipple—or 1 fluid oz before each feeding, (McIntyre, 2005); 1 cup daily for toddlers; see tea dosage guidelines for older children,

◇ **Tincture**: 10-30 drops up to 4 times/day,

*****

Chamomile:

Uses: Anxiety, teething, upset stomach, muscle and digestive spasms, nausea, colic

Research: Although the study had a very small sample size, the authors found that Chamomile (specifically, *Matricaria Chamomilla*) improved some symptoms of attention-deficit hyperactivity disorder.

Chamomile oil was highly active against clinically relevant acyclovir-resistant herpes simplex virus, type 1 strains.

Precautions: Avoid if allergic to daisy family (Asteraceae), including ragweed; anaphylaxis to Chamomile is well known, (Subiza, 1989; Reider, 2000); to avoid contamination, use only commercial preparations.

Dosage/Administration :

- ◇ **Capsule**: ½ **capsule** tid for 50-lb child

- ◇ **Tincture**: follow package directions or **10-30 drops**, up to qid,

- ◇ **Tea**: infant: **1-3 tsp**/day; toddler: ½ cup/day; 50-lb child: 1 cup tea or 1 dropperful extract/day

- ◇ **Tea**: colic: start slowly at 1 oz/day; watch for side effects before increasing to 3-4 oz/day

- ◇ **Topically** as a wash or salve,

Dandelion:

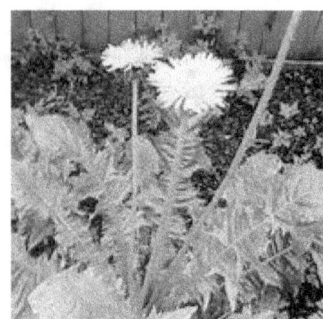

Uses: Internal: diuretic (bladder irritations), mild laxative, increases bile secretion (liver disorders) External: warts, (<u>White, 1998</u>), acne

Precautions: Do not use in children with acute gall bladder problems. Do not give to children allergic to the Asteraceae (formerly called Compositae) species (such as Chamomile, Yarrow root).

Dosage/Administration:

Fresh greens as a vegetable in season, can be steamed, or steamed and marinated

⬦ <u>Root tea</u>: ¼-1 cup daily or as a skin wash for acne,

⬦ <u>Tincture</u>: 10-15 drops 2-3 times daily.

⬦ Dandelion juice for warts: squeeze white juice from stems directly on wart several times/day for several weeks,

Echinacea:

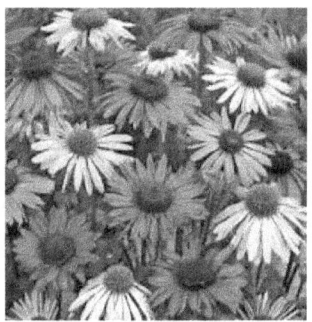

Uses:: Immune system support, childhood fevers, respiratory tract infections, (Cohen, 2004), Echinacea decreased the risk of subsequent colds, [Weber, 2005]), flu, sore throats and coughs; externally for wounds, eczema, chicken pox/herpes.

Research: Echinacea tincture stimulated T cells within 24 hours of ingestion,

Precautions: Not for use during immune disorders such as lupus, tuberculosis, multiple sclerosis, or HIV infection, rarely, patients with asthma, eczema, or hay fever have shown allergic reactions; not for children with allergy to Daisy family (Asteraceae); limit use to 10 days at a time, then take a 5-day break; for eczema (external use), take only a 2-day break. Do not give to children younger than 2 years of age.

Dosage/Administration:

- **Capsule/glycerite/tincture**: 50-lb child: 1 dropperful glyceride or tincture; 1 capsule,

- **Tincture**: ½ tsp bid to prevent colds and infections; for acute infections ½-1 tsp as often as every 2 hours (Romm, 2000); range from 1 drop/5 lbs body weight to 1 drop/1 lb body weight, depending on the condition's severity,

- For acute infections, ¼-½ tsp. every 2 hours; for chronic infections, 3 times/day,

- For skin infections, make a topical tincture of 1 teaspoon per ¼ cup water to use as a rinse,

- Tea: see tea dosage guidelines.

Elderberry:

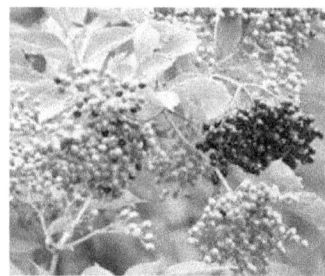

Uses: Fevers, stimulate the immune system, antiviral, flu, infections, asthma

Precautions: Use only blue-black elderberries; the red ones are toxic. Do NOT ingest the stem because of its cyanide content; do not use the leaves, roots, or bark internally. Only use cooked berries. Uncooked berries can cause nausea and vomiting. Large doses of elderberry juice can cause diarrhea.

Dosage/Administration:

- ◇   <u>Tea</u>: ½-1 cup up to qid, taken hot.

- ◇   <u>Prepared Syrup</u>: 1-2 tablespoons/day or 1-2 tsp up to tid.

To make syrup, use 1 cup fresh *or* ½ cup dried Elderberries, 3 cups water and 1 cup honey. Boil the berries in water, reduce heat and simmer 30-45 minutes. Smash the berries, strain them and add the honey to the strained liquid. Bottle and store in the refrigerator up to 2-3 months.

- ◇   <u>Tincture</u>: ¼-1 tsp up to 3 times/day.

*****

Eucalyptus:

Uses: Decongestant for coughs and chest infections

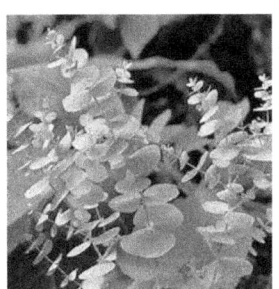

Precautions: Essential oil is *not* for internal use; internal use may cause seizures.

Child must be 2 yrs of age to use eucalyptus; do *not* apply to face of small children.

Not for patients with liver, gallbladder, or digestive diseases. Topical poisoning, although rare, has been reported.

Dosage/Administration

◇ **Chest rub:** dilute 0.5-2 ml eucalyptus oil in 25 ml almond oil, apply to chest or 1 drop per 5 ml sesame oil,

*****

Evening Primrose Oil:

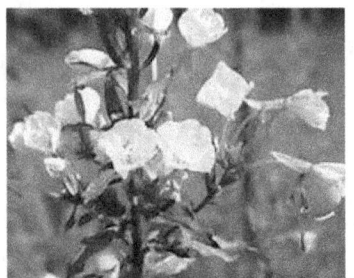

Uses: Eczema and atopic dermatitis, PMS, mastalgia, ADHD, ADHD with borderline zinc deficiency.

Precautions: May trigger temporal lobe epilepsy, especially in schizophrenics receiving phenothiazine's; side effects include nausea, stomach pain, and headache. Do not give to children who have a seizure disorder.

Dosage/Administration:

⋄ **Eczema**: 1-2 g/day from capsules, but not greater than 0.5 g/kg body weight daily.

⋄ **Mastalgia**: 3-4 g/day (1 g **tid-qid**) from capsules, (Integrative Medicine, 2000).

⋄ **PMS**: 3 g/day (1 g tid) from capsules, (Integrative Medicine, 2000).

Fennel

Uses: Upset stomach, gas, colic, cramps from diarrhea, to promote milk flow in nursing mothers

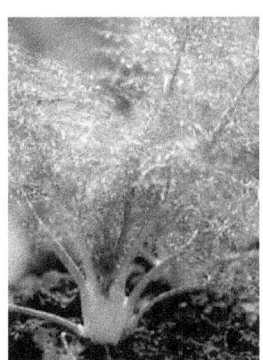

Precautions: Large doses may cause nausea, vomiting, and skin irritation; essential oil is *not* for infants or small children,). Long-term use may cause premature thelarche in children younger than 2 years.

Food allergy has been reported, although it is rare.

NOTE: Filling up infant on tea leaves less room for milk. *Do not substitute tea for milk or formula!*

Dosage/Administration:

- ⋄ **Infant colic**: 3-4 oz tea/day,

- ⋄ **Other conditions**: see tea dosage guidelines.

*****

Garlic

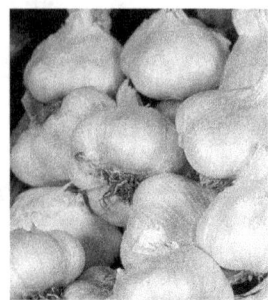

Uses: Respiratory infections, ear infections

Research/Future Possibilities: Garlic may increase oxygenation and improve dyspnea in children with hepatopulmonary syndrome. Garlic cloves have been used to eliminate warts, but caution is advised to avoid contact dermatitis. Constituents in garlic exhibit anticancer actions.

Precaution: Large quantities can irritate mouth or stomach, use sparingly for children younger than 2 years of age. May interact with drugs used to alter platelet function and coagulation.

CAUTION: Topical application can result in Garlic skin burns.

Dosage/Administration

♦   **Cooked**: children can eat rice or other foods flavored with Garlic or can eat ½-3 cloves daily

♦   **Garlic oil**: a 50-lb child can take ½ capsule Garlic oil several times a day with food

♦   **Tea**: see tea dosage guidelines; up to 4 cups daily can be used during colds

♦   **Syrup**: ½-1 tsp/day,

♦   **Supplements**: per package dosages

*****

Ginger:

Uses: Nausea, motion sickness, vomiting, digestive cramping, stomach upsets, muscle aches, menstrual cramps, headaches

Research: *Helicobacter pylori*, recognized as a primary etiologic factor in the development of gastritis and peptic ulcer disease, was susceptible in vitro to methanol extract of Ginger.

Precautions: Do not use during childhood fevers or in children with gallstones; in large doses over long periods, ginger can cause inflammation and weakness. Although a theoretical additive effect to Warfarin has not been investigated in humans, it may be best to avoid this combination.

Dosage/Administration:

◊ **Fresh herb/extract/capsule**: grate fresh Ginger into teas or follow package directions for extract or capsule,

◊ **Ginger root**: <3 yrs: 25 mg **qid**; 3-6 yrs: 50-75 mg **qid**; 7-11 yrs: 125 mg **qid**; ≤12 yrs: 250 mg **qid**,

◊ **Tea**: 2 slices Ginger in 1 cup water, see tea dosage guidelines

◊ **Tincture**: 5-25 drops in water up to 4 times/day

*****

Hops:

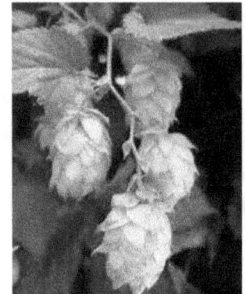

Uses: Restlessness, hyperactivity, insomnia, headaches, pain

Research/Future Possibilities: See Lemon Balm.

Precautions: Not for those with estrogen-dependent disorders; not appropriate in children with bedwetting, lethargy, or depression; not for long-term use; may cause skin irritation. There is a potential additive effect with drugs that sedate, such as anticonvulsants, antianxiety medications, and tricyclic antidepressants,

Dosage/Administration

◇ **Bath**: add a few drops of oil or dried herbs in a stocking to bath water,

*****

Hyssop:

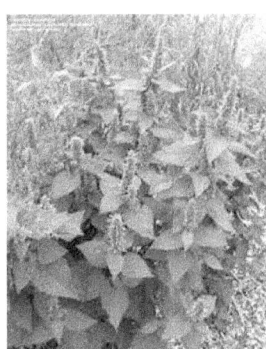

Uses: Coughing, colds and flu, chronic phlegm

Research/Future Possibilities: Muscle-relaxing activity of the essential oil has been shown on guinea pig and rabbit intestine.

Precautions: Do not give to children <2 yrs of age; use essential oil in very small quantities only for children.

Dosage/Administration:

    ◇   **Tea**: can be combined with Lemongrass and Elderberry as tea to treat childhood fevers; see <u>tea dosage guidelines.</u>

Juniper:

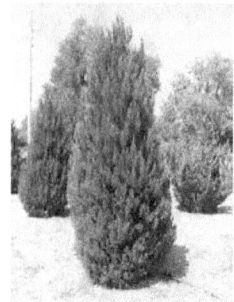

Uses: Diuretic, upset stomach, menstrual pain, urinary tract infection

Precautions: Do not give to children <2 yrs of age; contraindicated for those with kidney infection and inflammation,

NOTE: do not use longer than 4 wks because of potential kidney damage.

Dosage/Administration:

- ◇ <u>Menstrual pain</u>: use a weak tea of **15 g** berries in 500 ml water,

- ◇ <u>Urinary tract infection</u>: PO berry juice: dilute in water

- ◇ Other conditions: see <u>tea dosage guidelines</u>

*****

Lemon Balm:

Uses: Nervousness, anxiety, hyperactivity, sleep disorders, irritability, tension, antiviral

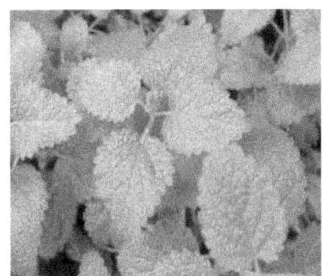

Research/Future Possibilities: Administration of Lemon Balm quelled laboratory-induced stress. Lemon Balm essential oil affected the infectivity of enveloped herpesviruses, an extract of Lemon Balm leaves inhibited replication of herpes simplex virus type 2,

Precautions: There is a potential additive effect with drugs that sedate, such as anti-convulsants, anti-anxiety medications, and tricyclic anti-depressants

Dosage/Administration:

- ◇   Infants ¼ **cup tid**

- ◇   Young children up to 50 lbs: up to **5 oz tid**

- ◇   <u>Older children</u>: **1-3 cups**/day

- ◇   <u>Tincture</u>: **¼-1 tsp** as needed

- ◇   <u>Cream</u>: topically as needed

- ◇   <u>Massage oil</u>: dilute **2-3 drops** per tablespoon of carrier oil

- ◇   Add a strong infusion to a warm bath

Lemongrass

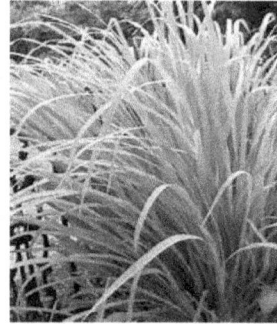

Uses: Childhood fevers

Precautions: None identified

Dosage/Administration:

⋄ **Tea**: use in tea with Hyssop and Elderberry; see <u>tea dosage guidelines.</u>

*****

Licorice:

Uses: Clears mucus from chest and upper respiratory tract, soothes inflammation in digestive tract and lungs

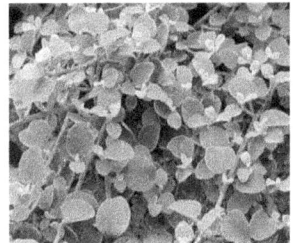

Precautions: Avoid Licorice if the child has high blood pressure or adrenal diseases.

Dosage/Administration:

- ◇ <u>Tincture</u>: **2 to 20 drops** up to 4 times daily. Start with the lowest dose; if not sufficient, it may be increased.

- ◇ <u>Decoction and infusion</u>: **⅓ of a teacup**. To make a Licorice decoction, add 1 tablespoon of chopped Licorice to 2 cups of boiling water for 20-30 minutes.

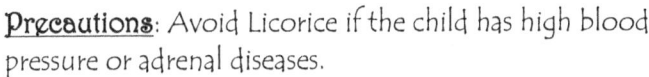

*****

Lobelia:

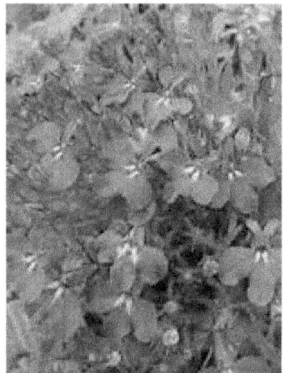

Uses: Expectorant, coughs, asthma

Precautions: Do not administer during shock or nervous prostration, low blood pressure or paralysis, or with dyspnea from heart disease; small quantities may cause slight nausea or a tight sensation in throat; give to children ≤5 yrs of age only; expect expectoration!

Do not use large doses.

Dosage/Administration:

◊ **Tea**: infuse no more than ¼ **tsp** dried herb/1 cup hot water; a 50-lb child can drink up to 1 cup **tid**,; see <u>tea dosage guidelines.</u>

*****

Nettle:

Uses: Allergies, hay fever, colds, coughs

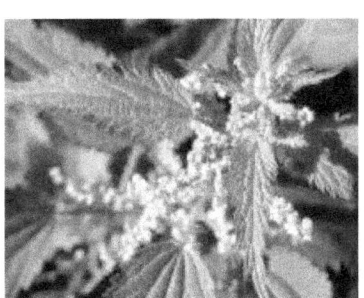

Precautions: Do not give to children <2 yrs of age; do not give to those with severe allergies, especially during anaphylactic shock; excessive use may interfere with these drugs: hypoglycemic, hyperglycemic, anti-diabetics, and central nervous system depressants.

Contact dermatitis can occur with fresh leaf.

Dosage/Administration:

⋄ **Capsule/tea**: a 50-lb child can have ½ capsule/day or ½ cup tea/day to begin, increasing to **tid** during allergy season; 2 "OO" size capsules 2 or 3 times daily; see tea dosage guidelines

⋄ **Tincture**: ¼–½ tsp up to 4 times/day.

⋄ **Cooked**: can serve as steamed fresh greens, but be careful of the Nettles; use gloves when gathering and preparing.

*****

Plantain:

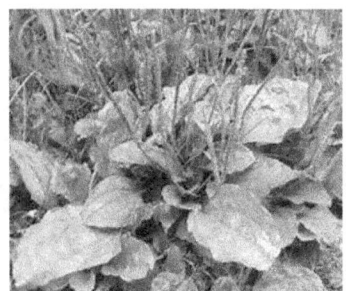

Uses: Externally for bee stings, poison oak or ivy rash, chicken pox, scrapes; internally for urinary tract inflammation, respiratory inflammation, or chronic cough.

Precautions: Internal use may cause nausea, vomiting, anorexia, flatus, diarrhea, bloating, or obstruction.

Dosage/Administration:

◇   **Tea** (internal): for urinary or lung disorders, make a tea of ½ tsp dried herb; administer as often as q2h,

◇   **Topical**: apply fresh poultice of leaves or apply leaves directly.

*****

Tea Tree Oil:

Uses: Acne, athlete's foot

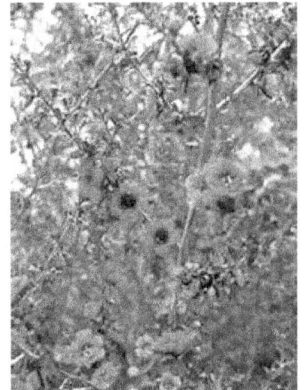

Research/Future Possibilities: Formulations containing tea tree oil were more active than soft soap as a hygienic skin wash against *Escherichia coli*. Application of 100% tea tree oil may have therapeutic benefit in nickel-induced contact hypersensitivity in human skin. Tea Tree Oil has been used successfully to treat warts in a pediatric patient.

Precautions: Oil may burn if it gets into eyes, nose, mouth, or tender areas. *Do not give internally*. Do not give to individuals allergic to Celery or Thyme because they share a potential allergen.

Dosage/Administration:

◇   Dilute for use in small children: **1-2 drops** per teaspoon of carrier oil, such as almond or olive,

◇   5% oil gel was used effectively on acne,

*****

Thyme:

Uses: Anti-inflammatory, coughs, bronchitis, upper respiratory mucus, sore throats, colic

Research/Future Possibilities: Thyme's essential oil has mosquito-repellent activity for hairless mice. Antifungal activity of the essential oil has been established. Essential oils exhibit antibacterial/antimicrobial activity.

Precautions: Never use essential oil internally or near eyes, nose, mouth, or sensitive mucous membranes. In large dosages can cause diarrhea. One case of allergy has been reported, cross reaction occurred within the Lamiae family, which includes Hyssop.

Dosage/Administration:

⋄   **Bath**: for infants, add strained tea to bath water,

⋄   **Chest rub**: add **10 drops** Thyme oil diluted in 20 ml Almond or Sunflower oil, or **5-10 drops** diluted with 2 tablespoons Almond oil for topical application.

⋄   **Tea**: see <u>tea dosage guidelines</u> or use **¼-1 cup** up to **tid**

⋄   **Tincture**: 10 drops to ½ tsp up to **tid**.

*****

Valerian:

Uses: Insomnia, dyssomnia, anxiety, hyperactivity, attention-deficit hyperactivity disorder, muscle or digestive cramps, flatulence, sleep difficulties in children with intellectual deficits.

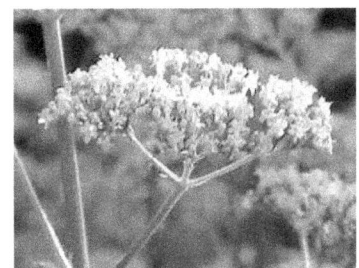

Precautions: For some children, Valerian can have a slight simulating effect—discontinue if this occurs, .

Withdrawal syndrome can occur after long-term use, can be mentally habit forming; in large doses (>100 g daily) can cause muscle pain and heart palpitations; may be **toxic** to liver when used for an extended period. There is a potential additive effect with drugs that sedate, such as anticonvulsants, anti-anxiety medications, and tricyclic anti-depressants.

Dosage/Administration:

- ◊ **Capsules**: Follow package directions

- ◊ **Tea/tincture**: See dosage guidelines

*****

Yarrow:

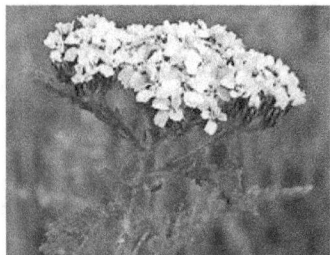

Uses: Externally for inflammatory skin conditions such as chicken pox, poison ivy and oak rashes; internally for fever, colds, and flu.

Research: Yarrow's antioxidant and anti-inflammatory effects have been confirmed. The extract of Yarrow exhibits a hepatoprotective effect, which may be partly attributed to its observed calcium channel blocking activity.

Precautions: Contraindicated for children allergic to daisy family, (Asteraceae).

Dosage/Administration:

⋄ **Tea**: see tea dosage guidelines

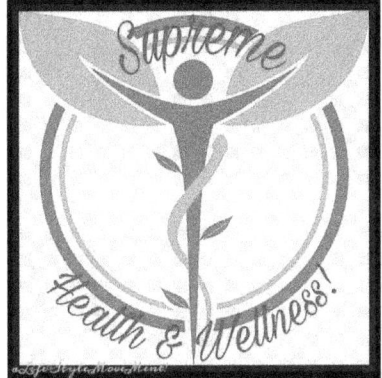

Four

Understanding Commercial Products

*****

Food Irradiation

Food Irradiation, also called 'cold Pasteurization' and is used in more than 40 countries to treat everything from frog legs to rice.

Irradiation exposes food to excessively high and un-natural doses of X-rays, Gamma Radiation, or High-Energy Electrons in-order to kill microbes and insects and in-activate Natural Enzymes that cause Natural Germination and Ripening of fruits and veggies.

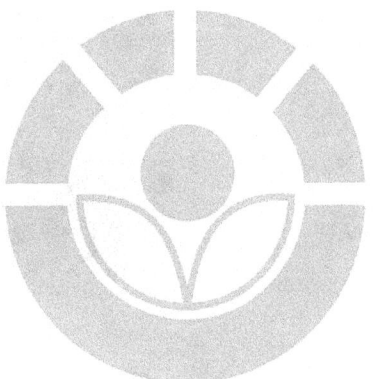

TREATED BY IRRADIATION

Because **irradiation** produces compounds that are not present in the original foods, it is treated as a food additive, and the level of radiation that may be used is regulated.

Irradiation- A process that exposes foods to Radiation in-order to kill contaminating organisms and retard the ripening and spoilage of fruits and vegetables.

Irradiated foods must be labeled with the *Radura* symbol shown above and the statement "*treated with radiation*" or "*treated by irradiation*."

The *Radura* symbol is **not** required on the labels of foods that contain Irradiated herbal elements, spices or other Irradiated ingredients.

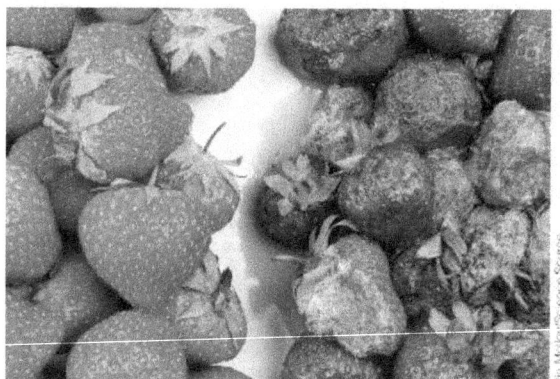

After 2 weeks in cold storage, the strawberries on the left, which were treated by Irradiation, remain free of mold, whereas the untreated strawberries on the right, which were picked at the same time, are covered with mold.

Food Packaging

*****

Packaging plays an important role in food preservation; it keeps molds and bacteria out, keeps moisture in, and protects food from physical damage. An open package of refrigerated cheddar cheese will be moldy in a few days, but an unopened package will stay fresh for weeks.

Food packaging is continually being improved. In the past two decades, for instance, consumer demand for fresh and easy-to-prepare foods has led manufacturers to offer partially cooked pasta, vegetables, seafood, fresh and cured meats, and dry products such as whole-bean and ground coffee in packaging that, if unopened, will keep perishable food fresh much longer than will conventional packaging.

Vacuum packaging and **Modified Atmosphere Packaging (MAP)** use plastics or other packaging materials that are impermeable to oxygen. In vacuum packaging, the air inside the package is removed prior to sealing in-order to eliminate the oxygen.

In Modified Atmosphere Packaging, *the air is flushed out and replaced with another Gas, such as Carbon Dioxide, Sodium Dioxide or Nitrogen.*

Both Carbon Dioxide and Sodium Dioxide are scientifically classified as Poison = TOXIC *when eaten!*

Carbon Dioxide is Human WASTE Product!

In both of these types of packaging, the low Oxygen level prevents the growth of Aerobic bacteria, slows the ripening of fruits and vegetables, and slows down Oxidation reactions, which cause discoloration in fruits and vegetables and rancidity in fats.

Modified Atmosphere Packaging (MAP)- A preservation technique used to prolong the shelf life of processed or fresh food by changing the gases surrounding the food in the package.

Packaging can protect food from spoilage, but even the best packaging can introduce risk if it becomes part of the food. A variety of substances found in paper and plastic containers and packaging, and even dishes, can leach into food.

Substances that are known to contaminate food are regulated by the EPA and the FDA. However, these regulations apply only to the *intended* use of the product.

When a product is used improperly, substances from its packaging can migrate into food. For instance, some plastics migrate into food when heated in a microwave oven. Thus, only containers designed for microwave cooking should be used for microwaving food.

This science underscores the need to grow our own food so that we can have direct access to Fresh Fruits and Veggies – Life Elements, WITHOUT the TOXIC packaging from commercial foods.

Bisphenol A from plastics

*****

Bisphenol A (BPA) is a chemical in plastic that's used in hard, transparent water bottles, baby bottles, and food containers as well as the coating *inside* canned food items.

Some but not all plastic containers marked with recycle codes 3 or 7 are made with BPA.

There is some concern that BPA could adversely affect development in fetuses, infants, and children.

The FDA supports efforts to eliminate the use of BPA in baby bottles and infant feeding cups and to replace BPA or minimize BPA levels in food can linings.

Aseptic processing

*****

The juice boxes that fit so conveniently into school lunch bags are produced by **Aseptic processing**. This technique heats foods to temperatures that result in Sterilization. The sterilized foods are then placed in sterilized packages, using sterilized packaging equipment. If the package remains unopened, juice and other aseptically packaged foods can remain free of microbial growth at room temperature for years.

Preservation techniques that rely on temperature benefit consumers by providing appealing, safe foods, but these foods are not risk free, particularly if they are handled incorrectly.

If foods are not heated long enough or to a high enough temperature, or if they are not kept cold enough, they could pose a risk of food-borne illness.

In addition, some types of cooking can generate hazardous chemical reactions.

Pesticides: Risks & Benefits

*****

Pesticides are used to prevent plant diseases and insect infestations. They are applied both to crops in the fields and to harvested produce in-order to prevent spoilage and extend shelf life. Crops that are grown using **pesticides** generally produce higher yields and look more appealing because they have less insect damage.

Once they have been applied, however, pesticides can travel into water supplies, soil, and other parts of the environment. Because pesticides enter the environment, pesticide residues are found not only on the treated plants but also in meat, poultry, fish, and dairy products.

The potential risks of pesticides to consumers depend on the size, age, and health of the person who consumes the pesticides and on the type and amount consumed.

To protect public health and the environment, the types of pesticides that may be used on food crops, the frequency of their use, and the amount of residue that may remain when foods reach consumers are regulated. The EPA approves and registers pesticides that are used in food production and establishes Tolerances.

Pesticide Tolerances are the maximum amounts of **pesticide** residues that may remain in or on a food. *To establish tolerances that are safe for both children and adults, the EPA considers tests done in experimental animals and on cells growing in the laboratory, as well as the amount of the* **pesticide** *to which consumers are likely to be exposed.* **Tolerances are then usually set at least 100 times lower than the highest dose that has no harmful effects in test animals.**

The FDA and the USDA monitor **pesticide** residues in foods. In general, pesticide residue levels in both domestic and imported foods have been found to be well below federally permitted limits.

These Tolerance levels that the FDA and USDA allow are broad, and intended to allow a specific number of people to become sick or die WITHOUT any repercussions to the manufacturer.

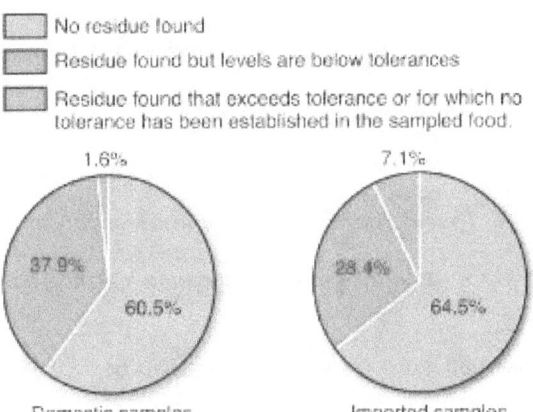

☐ No residue found
☐ Residue found but levels are below tolerances
☐ Residue found that exceeds tolerance or for which no tolerance has been established in the sampled food.

1.6%   37.9%   60.5%
Domestic samples

7.1%   28.4%   64.5%
Imported samples

Industrial Contaminants

*****

Industrial Chemicals that contaminate the environment ultimately find their way into the food supply. Especially given the scientific fact that NOTHING leaves the Earth. Fish accumulate substances from the water in which they live and feed. Shellfish accumulate contaminants because they feed by passing large volumes of water through their bodies. Pollutants in the water can also contaminate crops and move through the food chain into meat and milk.

One group of Carcinogenic Compounds that pollutes the environment is Poly-Chlorinated Biphenyls (PCBs). Prior to the 1970s, these chemicals were used in the manufacture of electrical capacitors and transformers, plasticizers, waxes, and paper. PCBs in runoff from manufacturing plants contaminated water, particularly near the Great Lakes.

PCBs are no longer produced, but because they do not degrade, they are still in the environment and accumulate in fish caught in contaminated waters. PCBs are a particular problem for pregnant and lactating women because prenatal exposure to PCBs and consumption of contaminated breast milk can damage the fetal and infant nervous system and cause learning deficits.

Pregnant and breastfeeding women should check with their local health department for recommendations regarding fish consumption.

Other contaminants from the manufacturing process include elements such as Chlordane (used to control termites); Radioactive Substances such as Strontium-90; and toxic metals such as Cadmium, Lead, Arsenic, and Mercury have found their way into fish and shellfish.

Cadmium and Lead can significantly impede or interfere with the absorption of other Minerals. Cadmium can cause kidney damage, and lead can impair brain development.

Arsenic is believed to increase the risk of cancer.

Mercury, which has been consistently been found in large fish, particularly swordfish, king mackerel, tilefish, and shark, damages nerve cells. Because Mercury is especially damaging during prenatal development, pregnant women are advised to avoid certain types of fish and limit their consumption of others

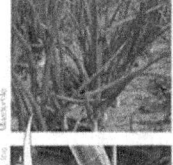
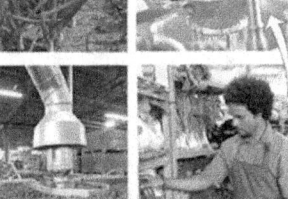
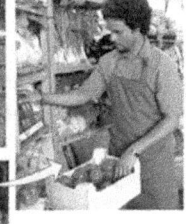

Farm Crops can be contaminated with bacteria before they are even harvested. Good agricultural practices help minimize contamination during growing, harvesting, sorting, packing, and storage.

Processing Contamination of processing equipment can transfer microbes to food. To prevent contamination, processors must follow guidelines concerning cleanliness and training of workers; develop a protocol that anticipates how biological, chemical, or physical hazards are most likely to occur; and establish appropriate measures to prevent them from occurring.

Transportation During transport, poor sanitation and inadequate refrigeration can contaminate food and allow microbes to grow. Clean containers and vehicles, plus refrigeration, can prevent the growth of food-borne bacteria.

Table Even a safe food can be contaminated in the home. Consumers can prevent food-borne illness at their table by carefully washing hands and food preparation equipment, as well as by handling, storing, and preparing food properly.

Retail Food can become contaminated during handling or storage in grocery stores or during preparation in restaurants. The FDA's Food Code provides recommendations for the handling and service of food in an effort to help owners and employees at retail establishments prevent food-borne illness. Local health inspections ensure cleanliness and proper procedures.

Chemicals used in agricultural production and industrial wastes contaminate the environment and can find their way into the food supply. *How harmful these chemicals are depends on whether they persist in the environment and whether they accumulate in the organisms that consume them or can be broken down and excreted by those organisms.*

Some of these contaminants are eliminated from the environment quickly because they are able to be broken down by micro-organisms or chemical reactions.

Others remain in the environment for very long periods, and when taken up by plants and small animals, they are not metabolized or excreted.

When these plants or small animals are consumed by larger animals that are in turn eaten by still larger animals, the contaminants accumulate, reaching higher concentrations at each level of the food chain. This process is called **Bio-accumulation.**

<u>*Because the toxins are not eliminated from the body, the greater the amount consumed, the greater the amount present in the body.*</u>

This un-natural process may be at the root-cause of several of the Health issues that are currently on the rise and that causes pre-mature death!

Bio-accumulation- The process by which compounds accumulate or build up in an organism faster than they can be broken down or excreted.

This is why it is paramount that if YOU haven't started your own Quality Food Supply = Garden......PLEASE STOP RIGHT NOW AND BEGIN!!!!!!!!

Abbreviations

*****

Ac .... *before meals*

Bid .... *2 times daily*

BUN .... *blood urea nitrogen*

CBC .... *complete blood cell count*

CNS .... *central nervous system*

DHEA .... *dehydroepiandrosterone*

ECG .... *electrocardiogram*

Er .... *extended release*

Gal .... *gallon*

GERD .... *gastroesophageal reflux disease*

GLA .... *Gamma Linolenic Acid*

HIV .... *Human Immunodeficiency Virus*

I&O .... Intake and Output

IgA .... Immunoglobulin A

IgG .... Immunoglobulin G

IgM .... Iimmunoglobulin M

In .... inch

IV .... intravenous

MAOI .... monoamine oxidase inhibitor

Mo .... month

NMDA .... N-methyl-D-aspartate

NNRTI .... nonnucleoside reverse transcriptase inhibitor

NSAID .... nonsteroidal antiinflammatory drug

OTC .... over the counter

Pc .... after meals

PMS .... premenstrual syndrome

PO .... by mouth

Pp .... postprandial (following a meal)

Prn .... as required

Q .... every

q2hr .... every 2 hours

q3hr .... every 3 hours

q4hr .... every 4 hours

q6hr .... every 6 hours

q12hr .... every 12 hours

qAM .... every morning

qd-bid .... 1-2 times daily

qhr .... every hour

qid4 .... times daily

qPM .... every night

qs .... sufficient quantity

Tbsp. .... tablespoon

tid3 .... times daily

tid-qid .... 3-4 times daily

tsp .... teaspoon

wk .... week

Abortifacient: An active ingredient/substance in a Herbal Element that induces abortion.

Aril: A botanical term used to denote an accessory seed coating that may form a fleshy, cuplike structure around the immature seed (ovule), as in yew and nutmeg. The aril is often brightly colored and edible.

Binomial: The unique, two-part scientific name used to identify a plant. The first name is the genus; the second, the species. A designation of the variety may also follow to further differentiate the plant. Because common names differ from region to region and a single common name may often denote several herbs that differ widely from each other, use of the binomial is the only reliable way to accurately specify a particular herb.

Concentration: A means of expressing the amount of herb and solvent used in formulating an herbal preparation. For example, a tincture with a 1:5 concentration contains 1 part of the herb in grams to 5 parts of the solvent in milliliters. Concentration is not the same thing as potency (see <u>Potency</u>).

Crude herb: The raw plant, before it is dried and processed.

Decoction: A liquid preparation made by boiling plant parts (such as bark, roots, or rhizome) in water.

Diaphoretic: An element that increases/enhances diaphoresis – profuse perspiration and/or sweating.

Diuretic: An element or substance that promotes diuresis – the production of urine.

Expectorant: Medicinal element that promotes the secretion of sputum by the air passages.

Extract: A concentrated form of the herb that is derived when the crude herb is mixed with water, alcohol, or another solvent and distilled or evaporated. Extracts may be either fluid or solid.

Gall: A lump or ball that forms most often on the stems, leaves, or roots of plants at the sites of injuries caused by insects, fungi, bacteria, or other organisms. An example is the oak gall, which contains tannin.

Herbal Element: A plant that is used for its medicinal purposes. (This differs from the biological definition of an herb as a plant with no woody above-ground parts.)

Infusion: A liquid preparation made by pouring water over plant parts (such as dried or fresh leaves, flowers, or fruits) and allowing the mixture to steep. Hot water (below the boiling point) is usually used, but cold water may also be used. Making a cup of herbal tea is an example.

Minim: A fluid measure constituting 1/60; of a fluidrachm, which itself is about a teaspoonful (⅛ of a fluid ounce). A minim is about the equivalent of one drop of water.

Nutraceutical: A food that is used for its medicinal properties.

Oil, essential: The aromatic volatile oils extracted from various parts of the fresh herb. Essential oils are usually diluted before being used therapeutically.

Oil, infused: A mixture composed of the volatile oils of an herb and another oil. The so-called "carrier oil" is used to extract the volatile oils by soaking plant parts in it for a specified period.

Pharmacognosy: The study of chemicals taken from natural sources to be used as drugs or in the preparation of drugs. Sources may include plants, animals, or other life forms such as fungi, molds, and yeasts.

Phytochemical: The active chemical components, or constituents, present in a plant that account for its medicinal properties.

Phytoestrogen: Plant-derived xenoestrogens not generated from the endocrine system, but consumed from eating phytoestrogenic plants.

Phytomedicine: The use of plants, plant parts, and preparations made from them to prevent, treat, or cure various health conditions.

Phytotherapy: The use of medicinal plants to heal and restore balance.

Potency: A measure of the strength of the active chemical components contained in an herb or herbal preparation. Standardized products ensure that the consumer receives a dosage containing a consistent potency.

Poultice: Plant material (such as crushed fresh herbs) that has been wrapped in gauze or similar soft cloth, moistened, and applied topically.

Powder: The dried product of an extraction process during which the herb is distilled, using a solvent such as alcohol or water, after which the solvent is completely removed. The dry solid that remains either is already in powder form or may be ground into it.

Rhizome: An underground plant stem, growing more or less horizontally, that usually has roots on its underside and bears buds.

Tincture: A plant extract made by soaking herbs in a liquid (such as water, alcohol, vinegar, or glycerine) for a specified period, then straining and discarding the plant material. The remaining liquid is used therapeutically. Tinctures typically are made at a concentration of 1:5 to 1:10.

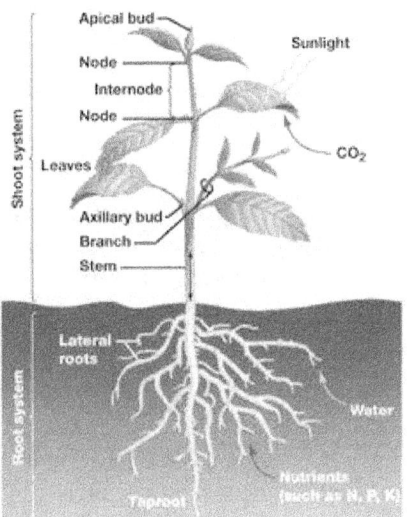

Herbal Resources:

******

The following are the online resources that provide current, reliable information about herbal elements and products, their uses, and their health effects. Some are consumer oriented, and others are intended for health professionals. The names of the sponsoring organizations' home pages are arranged alphabetically. URLs are provided for each individual site, or for the Internet portal through which the site may be accessed.

AGRICOLA (AGRICultural OnLine Access): http://agricola.nal.usda.gov/

Alternative Medicine Home Page, from the University of Pittsburgh: http://www.pitt.edu/~cbw/altm.html

American Botanical Council: http://abc.herbalgram.org/site/PageServer?pagename=Homepage

American Herbalists Guild: http://www.americanherbalistsguild.com/

American Herbal Pharmacopoeia: http://www.herbal-ahp.org/

American Holistic Health Association: http://www.ahha.org

American Holistic Medical Association: http://www.holisticmedicine.org

American Holistic Nurses Association: http://www.ahna.org

American Society of Pharmacognosy: http://www.phcog.org/

Association of Natural Medicine Pharmacists: http://www.anmp.org

British Herbal Medicine Association: http://www.bhma.info/

Christopher Hobbs Virtual Herbal: http://www.christopherhobbs.com/

Dr. Duke's Phytochemical and Ethnobotanical Databases, from the Agricultural Research Service: http://www.ars-grin.gov/duke/plants.html

European Herbal & Traditional Medicine Practitioners Association:
http://www.ehpa.eu/

European Scientific Cooperative on Phytotherapy (ESCOP):
http://www.escop.com/

Herb Research Foundation (HRF): http://www.herbs.org

Herbal Medicine, from Medline Plus:
http://www.nlm.nih.gov/medlineplus/herbalmedicine.html

Herbs for Health, from About.com: http://altmedicine.about.com/

International Herb Association: http://www.iherb.org/

Rocky Mountain Herbal Institute: http://www.rmhiherbal.org/

RxList Alternatives: http://www.rxlist.com/script/main/art.asp?articlekey=78831

Southwest School of Botanical Medicine:
http://www.swsbm.com/HOMEPAGE/HomePage.html

United Plant Savers (UpS): http://unitedplantsavers.org/

United States Pharmacopoeia (USP): http://www.usp.org/

References:

LE Arnold, SM Pinkham, N Votolato: Does zinc moderate essential fatty acid and amphetamine treatment of attention deficit hyperactivity disorder?. *J Child Adolesc Psychopharmacol.* **100**(2), 2000, 111–117.

PA Balch: In *Prescription for Herbal Healing.* 2000, Avery, New York.

B Barrett: Efficacy and safety of Echinacea in treating upper respiratory tract infections in children: a randomized controlled trial. *J Pediatr.* **145**(1), 2004, 135–136.

EM Basch, CE Ulbricht: In *Natural Standard Herb & Supplement Handbook.* 2005, Mosby, St. Louis.

B Becker, U Kuhn, B Hardewig-Budny: Double-blind, randomized evaluation of clinical efficacy and tolerability of an apple pectin-chamomile extract in children with unspecific diarrhea. *Arzneimittelforschung.* **56**(6), 2006, 387–393.

M Benito, G Jorro, C Morales, A Pelaez, A Fernandez: Labiatae allergy: systemic reactions due to ingestion of oregano and thyme. *Ann Allergy Asthma Immunol.* **76**(5), 1996, 416–418.
JL Berdonces: Attention deficit and infantile hyperactivity. *Rev Enferm.* **24**(1), 2001, 11–14.

F Brinker: In *Herb contraindications and drug interactions.* 1998, Eclectic Medical, Sandy, Ore.

J Brush, E Mendenhall, A Guggenheim, et al.: The effect of *Echinacea purpurea, Astragalus membanaceus* and *Glycyrrhiza glabra* on CD69 expression and immune cell activation in humans. *Phytother Res.* **20**(8), 2006, 687–695.

PR Burkhard, K Burkhardt, CA Haenggeli, T Landis: Plant-induced seizures: reappearance of an old problem. *J Neurol.* **246**(8), 1999, 667–670.

WS Choi, BS Park, SK Ku, SE Lee: Repellent activities of essential oils and monoterpenes against Culex pipiens pallens. *J Am Mosq Control Assoc.* **18**(4), 2002, 348–351.

YK Chou, HJ Chen, MR Shaio, YM Kuo: In vitro antibiotic susceptibility of lactobacilli isolated from commercial products containing active lactobacilli. *Acta Paediatr Taiwan.* **45**(3), 2004, 141–144.

HA Cohen, I Varsano, E Kahan, EM Sarrell, Y Uziel: Effectiveness of an herbal preparation containing Echinacea, propolis, and vitamin C in preventing respiratory tract infections in children: a randomized, double-blind, placebo-controlled, multicenter study. *Arch Pediatr Adolesc Med.* **158**(3), 2004, 217–221.

T Darben, B Cominos, CT Lee: Topical eucalyptus oil poisoning. *Australas J Dermatol.* **39**(4), 1998, 265–267.

GW Elmer, LV McFarland: Biotherapeutic Agents in the Treatment of Infectious Diarrhea. *Gastroenterol Clin N Am.* **30**(3), 2001, 837–854.

A Fabio, C Cermelli, G Fabio, P Nicoletti, P Quaglio: Screening of the antibacterial effects of a variety of essential oils on microorganisms responsible for respiratory infections. *Phytother Res.* **21**(4), 2007, 374–377.

AJ Francis, RJ Dempster: Effect of valerian, Valeriana edulis, on sleep difficulties in children with intellectual deficits: randomised trial. *Phytomedicine.* **9**(4), 2002, 273–279.
A Fugh-Berman: Herbal Supplements: Indications, clinical concerns, and safety. *Nutrition Today.* **37**, 2002, 122–124.

P Gardiner, L Dvorkin, KJ Kemper: Supplement use growing among children and adolescents. *Pediatr Ann.* **33**(4), 2004, 227–232.

P Gardiner, KJ Kemper: Herbs in Pediatric and Adolescent Medicine. *Pediatrics in Review.* **21**(2), 2000, 44–57.

Gladstar R: *Family Herbal: A Guide to Living Life with Energy, Health and Vitality.* Storey, 2001.

RD Goldman, AL Rogovik, D Lai, S Vohra: Potential interactions of drug-natural health products and natural health products-natural health products among children. *J Pediatr*. **152**(4), 2008, 521–526.

S Gouin, H Patel: Unusual cause of seizure. *Pediatr Emerg Care*. **12**(4), 1996, 298–300.

R Harkness, S Bratman: In *Drug-Herb-Vitamin Interactions Bible*. 2

TABLE 22A-1 Summary of Top 25 Herbs

'e | 120

Herb	Common uses	Activity	Adverse effects and contraindications	Doses	Drug interactions
Aloe vera—*Aloe vera*	Orally—constipation, ulcerative colitis, gastroesophageal reflux, gastritis, peptic ulcer disease. Topically—psoriasis, minor cuts and burns	Orally, the anthraquinone has powerful cathartic properties. Also has antibacterial, antifungal, and antioxidant properties.	Abdominal pain and cramps Long-term use or abuse can cause diarrhea, weight loss, albuminuria, hematuria, and potassium depletion.	Orally, 100-200 mg aloe or 50 mg aloe extract daily Topically, 0.5% aloe extract cream applied to area TID	Caution in patients on digoxins; prolonged use can lead to hypokalemia.
Bilberry—*Vaccinium myrtilus*	Diabetic and hypertensive retinopathy	Flavonoid complex (anthocyanoside)		160 mg BID for retinopathy	
Black cohosh—*Cimicifuga racemosa*	Menopausal symptoms (hot flashes) and mood disturbances	Estrogen-like effects without estrogenic activity	GI upset, rash, headache, dizziness. Avoid in patients with hepatitis, breast cancer	Remifemin 20 mg tablet BID	No well-known drug interactions
Cranberry—*Vaccinium macrocarpon*	UTI prevention, urinary deodorizer	Proanthocyanidins seem to interfere with bacterial adherence to urinary tract epithelial cells. Mild antiinflammatory, antiplatelet, and antitumor effects	Excessive use (greater than 1 L daily) over a prolonged period of time could lead to uric acid kidney stone formation	One 8-oz glass daily	Daily ingestion of 250 ml cranberry juice can increase serum and urine salicylate level
Echinacea—*Echinacea angustifolia*	Decrease symptoms of common cold, diminishes recurrence of vaginal yeast infections	Immune stimulant	Nausea, abdominal pain, diarrhea, and vomiting Caution in patients with autoimmune disorders	A tablet of 300 mg of Echinacea dosed as 1 or 2 tablets TID	Theoretically can interfere with immunosuppressant medications
Elderberry—*Sambucus nigra*	Influenza	Antioxidant, antiinflammatory, and immunomodulating effects		Adult 15 ml QID for 3-5 days, child's dose is 15 ml (1 tablespoon) twice daily	
Evening primrose oil—*Oenothera biennis*	Mastalgia, osteoporosis, atopic dermatitis, neuropathy	gamma-linoleic acid (GLA)—antiinflammatory properties, possible antiestrogenic effects	Avoid in patients taking phenothiazines	3-4 g daily	Can potentiate effects of antiplatelet/anticoagulant drugs
Garlic—*Allium sativum*	Hypertension, atherosclerosis, prevention of stomach and colon cancer Topical treatment of dermal fungal infections (tinea corporis, tinea cruris, and tinea pedis)	Pharmacological effects attributed to allicin, ajoene, and other organosulfur constituents such as S-allyl-L-cysteine	Orally: breath and body odor, mouth and GI burning or irritation, heartburn, flatulence, nausea, vomiting, and diarrhea Topically: dermatitis, eczema, blisters, and scarring	Fresh garlic (1-2 cloves) daily, garlic extract (200-400 mg) BID to TID, topical garlic constituent ajoene at 0.4% cream, 0.6% gel, and 1.0% gel for the treatment of tinea	May potentiate effects of antiplatelet/anticoagulant drugs May decrease concentrations of INH and HIV medications
Ginger—*Zingiber officinale*	Morning sickness, motion sickness, nausea/vomiting, arthritis	Antiemetic, antiinflammatory, antihypertensive, antiplatelet, antipyretic, and antitussive properties	Rare: abdominal discomfort, heartburn, diarrhea, and a pepper-like irritant effect in the mouth and throat	250 mg QID prn for morning sickness, 500-1000 mg 30 min before travel for motion sickness, 500-1000 mg BID-TID for arthritis	Theoretically ginger can potentiate the effects of antiplatelet and anticoagulant drugs
Ginkgo—*Ginkgo biloba*	Age-related memory impairment, improving cognitive function, dementia, diabetic retinopathy, glaucoma, intermittent claudication, PMS, Raynaud syndrome, vertigo, tinnitus, sexual dysfunction related to SSRIs	Antioxidant, free radical scavenger Inhibits platelet aggregation Protects cell membranes, erythrocytes, neurons, and retinal tissue	Mild GI upset, headache, dizziness, palpitations, constipation, and allergic skin reactions Rare cases of spontaneous bleeding and seizures	120-240 mg divided TID	Can potentiate effects of antiplatelet/anticoagulant drugs

Herb	Uses	Action/Components	Side effects	Dosage	Drug interactions
Ginkgo—*Ginkgo biloba*	Age-related memory impairment, improving cognitive function, dementia, diabetic retinopathy, glaucoma, intermittent claudication, PMS, Raynaud syndrome, vertigo, tinnitus, sexual dysfunction related to SSRIs	Antioxidant, free radical scavenger Inhibits platelet aggregation Protects cell membranes, erythrocytes, neurons, and retinal tissue	Mild GI upset, headache, dizziness, palpitations, constipation, and allergic skin reactions Rare cases of spontaneous bleeding and seizures	120-240 mg divided TID	Can potentiate effects of antiplatelet/anticoagulant drugs
Ginseng—*Panax ginseng*	Adaptogen, improving cognition, nourishing stimulant, aphrodisiac Treatment of diabetes Treatment of erectile dysfunction and premature ejaculation	Ginsenosides or panaxosides	Adverse effects and contraindications—generally well tolerated, most common side adverse effect is insomnia	200-500 mg daily For erectile dysfunction 900 mg TID	None known to exist, but there are several potential theoretical drug interactions
Grape seed—*Vitis vinifera*	Venous insufficiency, ocular stress, atherosclerosis, hypertension	Antioxidant, vasodilating, antilipoperoxidant, and antiplatelet effects		360-720 mg daily	Induces cytochrome P450 and may decrease plasma levels of common prescription drugs such as warfarin, clopidogrel, and propranolol
Green tea—*Camellia sinensis*	Improve cognitive performance	Caffeine, catechins (antiinflammatory, antioxidant, and antimutagenic effects)	Nausea, vomiting, dyspepsia, dizziness, insomnia, tremors, restlessness, confusion	3 cups daily	Can potentiate effects of other CNS stimulants (amphetamines, cocaine, ephedrine)
Hawthorn—*Crataegus monogyna*	Chronic heart failure	Increases myocardial contractility, lengthens myocardial refractory period, increases coronary blood flow, increases cardiac output, and reduces oxygen consumption	Rare side effects include vertigo, dizziness, nausea, GI complaints, fatigue, sweating, rash, palpitations, headache, dyspnea, nosebleeds, sleeplessness, and agitation	80-300 mg TID of standardized hawthorn leaf with flower extract	Theoretical additive effects with beta-blockers, calcium channel blockers, digoxin, nitrates, and phosphodiesterase inhibitors
Horny goat weed—*Epimedium grandiflorum*	Sexual dysfunction, osteoporosis	Flavonoids, phytoestrogens	Dizziness, vomiting, dry mouth, thirst, and nosebleed Isolated case of hypotension	Unclear	
Horse chestnut seed—*Aesculus hippocastanum*	Chronic venous insufficiency, varicose veins, hemorrhoids	Permeability of venous capillaries and constricts veins	Dizziness, nausea, headache, and pruritus	300 mg horse chestnut seed extract BID	Theoretically can potentiate effects of antiplatelet and anticoagulant drugs
Kava kava—*Piper methysticum*	Anxiety, social anxiety disorder	Attributed to the kavalactones, which have anxiolytic, sedative, anticonvulsant, spasmolytic, antiinflammatory, and analgesic properties	Concern about potential hepatotoxicity has caused it to be banned from several countries, including Germany	100 mg TID (100 mg—standardized to contain 70% kavalactones)	Caution should to taken to avoid use with CNS depressants such as benzodiazepines, alcohol, and barbiturates
Milk thistle—*Silybum marianum*	Type 2 diabetes, alcohol-induced liver damage, and hepatitis B or C infection	Silymarin; antioxidant, free radical scavenger, inhibitor of lipid peroxidation, TNF inhibitor Decreases insulin resistance		Silymarin 200 mg TID	Might inhibit cytochrome P450
Olive leaf—*Olea europaea*	Hyperlipidemia, hypertension Prevention of CAD, osteoarthritis, rheumatoid arthritis	Antiinflammatory, antiplatelet, antioxidant effects		2-3 tablespoons daily added to diet	
Red clover—*Trifolium pratense*	Hot flashes, menopausal symptoms, hyperlipidemia	Contains isoflavones, acts as an alternative	Myalgia, headache, nausea, vaginal spotting	40-160 mg daily of standardized extract, 1-2 tsp dried flowers to make a cup of tea, or 2-4 ml of tincture TID	Theoretical interactions with birth control pills, estrogen replacement hormonal products, tamoxifen, blood thinners, and diabetes medications

Herb	Uses	Mechanism	Side Effects	Dosage	Drug Interactions
Saw palmetto—*Serenoa repens*	BPH, alopecia	Antiandrogenic, antiproliferative, and antiinflammatory	Dizziness, headache, nausea, vomiting, constipation. One case report of excessive bleeding during surgery - ? anti-platelet effect	160 mg BID or 320 mg once daily for BPH	Theoretically can potentiate effects of antiplatelet/anticoagulant drugs
Soy—*Glycine max*	Hyperlipidemia, menopausal symptoms, osteoporosis, cardiovascular disease	Contains phytoestrogens, known as isoflavones and lignans. Rich in calcium, iron, potassium, amino acids, vitamins, and fiber	May cause endometrial hyperplasia.	20-100 g daily of soy protein; 50-120 mg daily of concentrated soy isoflavones	Tofu and soy sauce contain tyramine—avoid with MAOIs. Can interfere with absorption of oral thyroid hormone replacement
St. John's Wort—*Hypericum perforatum*	Depression, somatization disorder, menstrual symptoms	Inhibits reuptake of serotonin, dopamine, and norepinephrine	Insomnia, vivid dreams, restlessness, anxiety, agitation, irritability, and mild GI complaints	300 mg TID	Multiple drug interactions, probably because it is a potent inducer of cytochrome P450. Can decrease levels of common important drugs (digoxin, OCPs, phenobarbital, phenytoin, and cyclosporine, etc.) Can also potentiate serotonin effects when taken with other SSRIs, meperidine, tramadol)
Valerian—*Valeriana officinalis*	Insomnia, anxiety	GABA agonist		400-900 mg taken up to 2 hours before bedtime	Can theoretically potentiate effects of other CNS depressants such as benzodiazepines, alcohol, and opiates
Yohimbe—*Pausinystalia yohimbe*	Erectile dysfunction, sexual dysfunction	MAO-inhibiting, calcium channel–blocking, and peripheral serotonin receptor–blocking effects	Excitation, tremor, insomnia, anxiety, hypertension, tachycardia, dizziness, gastric intolerance, salivation, sinusitis, irritability, headache, urinary frequency, fluid retention, rash, nausea, and vomiting. Avoid in patients with coronary artery disease, hypertension, BPH, anxiety	15-30 mg daily	Can potentiate MAOIs, TCAs, phenothiazenes, and stimulant drugs. Also antagonizing effects with antihypertensive drugs

Supreme Health & Fitness by Sean Ali!

Achieving and Maintaining Supreme Health by increasing the level of

Knowledge and Science of Life!

www.ingramcontent.com/pod-product-compliance
Lightning Source LLC
Chambersburg PA
CBHW081301170526
45165CB00011B/3364